Kathrin Braun (ed.)
Between Self-Determination and Social Technology

body cultures

Kathrin Braun (ed.)

Between Self-Determination and Social Technology
Medicine, Biopolitics and the New Techniques of Procedural Management

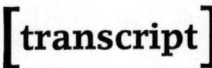

Bibliographic information published by the Deutsche Nationalbibliothek
The Deutsche Nationalbibliothek lists this publication in the Deutsche Nationalbibliografie; detailed bibliographic data are available in the Internet at http://dnb.d-nb.de

© 2011 transcript Verlag, Bielefeld

All rights reserved. No part of this book may be reprinted or reproduced or utilized in any form or by any electronic, mechanical, or other means, now known or hereafter invented, including photocopying and recording, or in any information storage or retrieval system, without permission in writing from the publisher.

Cover layout: Kordula Röckenhaus, Bielefeld
Typeset by Andreas Sturm
Printed by Majuskel Medienproduktion GmbH, Wetzlar
ISBN 978-3-8376-1747-4

Global distribution outside Germany, Austria and Switzerland:

Transaction Publishers
New Brunswick (U.S.A.) and London (U.K.)

Transaction Publishers   Tel.: (732) 445-2280
Rutgers University   Fax: (732) 445-3138
35 Berrue Circle   for orders (U.S. only):
Piscataway, NJ 08854   toll free 888-999-6778

Contents

Preface by William Ray Arney | 7

Between self-determination and social technology. Medicine, biopolitics and the new techniques of procedural management
An introduction
Kathrin Braun | 11

From social care to planning childbirth in the Federal Republic of Germany 1950-1975
Marion Schumann | 31

Planning death: Debates on euthanasia, end of life care and living wills in Germany since the 1970s
Isabella Jordan | 65

Genetic counseling and the fiction of choice: Taught self-determination as a new technique of social engineering
Silja Samerski | 95

Shifting responsibilities in the medical field: US-American bioethics and its move into the hospital setting
Helen Kohlen | 127

A speaking cure for conflicts: problematization, discourse stimulation and the ongoing of scientific 'progress'
Svea Luise Herrmann | 159

Post-apocalyptic discourse and the new modesty: governing preimplantation genetic diagnosis in the UK
Kathrin Braun and Susanne Schultz | 189

Is everything in good health?
From bio to nano—the proliferation of governmental ethics in France
Sabine Könninger | 215

New biopolitics? The articulation of demographic aims and gender policies in international population programs
Susanne Schultz | 239

List of Contributors | 271

Preface

We're free. That's the message in a bottle that floated off from the Movements of the 1960s. People who know themselves to be free people can stop unjust wars, win the vote for those excluded from democratic practices and full social participation, and reduce the power of people who had claimed authority on the basis of technical expertise.

Restructuring the medical encounter became emblematic of the possibilities of a freer life in institutions. The women's movement in particular took aim at the godlike physician—the doctor who, in the best interests of his patients, decided what needed to be done and did it, but who, also in the interest of his patients, did not speak—and toppled him. Armed with information and supported by free and open talk among friends and colleagues, women—eventually, all patients—demanded and won a seat at the medical decision-making table. The victors asserted that the power of medical authorities had been properly reduced or that, at least, power had come to be shared between interested parties.

Beginning around 1970 the structure of the medical encounter changed. Very quickly, medicine adopted the principle of informed consent, which was premised on the notion that a patient had to be told all the facts of her situation and all options for treatment so that she, not the physician, could be the principal decision maker about what medicine could do to her body, herself. Medical ethics was no longer just an internal code by which physicians might regulate themselves but became subject to public discussion about the proper role, place and function of physicians. Medical practices became matters of public policy. Medicine's object, the disease, the disability and the body that carried It, became a subject, a She or a He, a person who spoke, contended, thought, desired, felt, a person who angered, experienced pain, who changed, who wondered not just how, objectively, one dies but what it means to die, and what it means to live. People, especially free ones, are messier than objectified, medicalized bodies. Medicine changed to accommodate "the patient as a person."[1]

But now we have this remarkable collection of thoughtful empirical studies of the structure of medical practice that should make us wonder if, almost a half century after the Movements, we are truly free. Ranging from the intimacy of the genetic counseling session through the knot of legalities that emerge as we move from the human condition of "having to die" to the medico-legal problems of "planning my death" and on up to the level of National Ethics Committees and Boards, these studies paint a challenging, even perverse image of this so-called free individual. The new subject of medical practice not only *can* talk; she *must* talk. She not only is capable of making decisions; she must follow medicine-designed decision-making procedures, "social technologies that … avoid disruption, absorb disturbances, and allow for things to smoothly go on." At the national level citizens must engage in debates about ethics because public debate is *the solution* to ethically conflicted problems; public debate gives people a sense of participation in political discussions, but the discussions are socially designed so they do not interfere with the progress of science. We're not free. We revel in thinking that we are, but in fact we are well managed. We can say anything as long as we stick to the script, the preformed guidelines for proper speech. We're free as long as we don't say or do anything that matters.

This volume details how our interactions with modern medicine, public officials and with one another have been structured and refined to make us behave. New procedures forbid real talk, real conflict, any form of immoderation, silence, all the juiciness and earthiness of our humanity out of which the Movements flowered. We cannot disrupt scientific progress by

---

1   The first chapter of Tinsley Harrison's new medical textbook, Principles of Internal Medicine, was "The Patient as a Person." This was the first time medicine had thought of the patient as a person. Harrison's revolutionary manifesto said, in part, "the art of medicine is not confined to organic disease; it deals also with the mind of the patient and with his behavior as a thinking, feeling human being" (Harrison 1950, 4). It is worth noting that this was published in 1950, ten to twenty years before the revolutions of the Movements.

doing, as Bill McKibben put it, "an unlikely thing: we need to survey the world we now inhabit and declare it good. Good enough" (McKibben 2003, 109). Were we able to start there, we might imaginably push on toward the recovery of the Enlightenment ideal that "the only ethical human condition is the mutual, shared, respectful, civic recognition of human interdependence" (White 2004, 163). We would not spend our time talking with genetics expert trained to speak only in risk probabilities; we could find friends with whom to talk about how best to live in the great hope of expecting a baby. We would not wrap ourselves in the expert-granted "personal autonomy" to make, in advance, personal decisions about "my death" and fuss over the details of our living wills and final instructions; I could reflect on "my trust in my relatives and others around me, my faith that they will do what is right, [on the fact] that I can feel cared for as a human being".[2] I probably would not worry about the details of research on stem cell lines, pre-implantation diagnosis, or the latest efforts to control population growth; I might join with others to imagine what liberation, equality, enfranchisement and the like might mean in these times. A world that we declare "good enough" in scientific terms has a chance of being better in human terms.

This book says, "We're not really free, but we could try to be". It's a generous invitation.

WILLIAM RAY ARNEY
FRIDAY HARBOR

REFERENCES

Harrison, Tinsley (1950): Principles of internal medicine, Philadelphia, PA: The Blakiston Company.
McKibben, Bill (2003): Enough: Staying human in an engineered age, New York, NY: Henry Holt.
White, Curtis (2004): The middle mind: Why Americans don't think for themselves, New York, NY: HarperCollins.

---

2 From "Planning Death," this volume.

Between self-determination and social technology. Medicine, biopolitics and the new techniques of procedural management
An introduction

KATHRIN BRAUN

Doctor's attitudes toward patients are terribly condescending, especially toward women. You aren't supposed to read the record of your own body, and you are scolded like a child if you do. Doctors withhold information that you are dying. They withhold information that you might have a difficult pregnancy or childbirth. In playing God, their attitude is that you must have complete confidence in them to make all of your decisions for you. Why should they make your decisions?
(Boston Women's Health Collective 1970: 182)

Forty years have passed since a group of women, who called themselves "the doctors group", published the first edition of Our Bodies, Ourselves. What angered them was the experience of a double silence; the silence of doctors toward them, as denounced in the quote above, but also the experience of being silenced, of not being entitled to speak about their own bodily experience, not being taken seriously, and not being listened to. The first silence was one rife with knowledge and hubris: knowledge withheld from those whom it intimately concerned. Doctors, the women felt, were withholding knowledge about a patient's body, pregnancy, or imminent death, knowledge deemed too complicated and dangerous for those whom it concerned. Decision-making was left to those who could deal with that knowledge and who knew what they were doing, namely, the doctors. On the other side, there was a silence rife with ignorance and shame: ignorance that prevented them from posing questions, discussing options and insisting on making their own decisions, and shame about menstruation, masturbation, unwanted pregnancies, illegal abortions, post-partem depressions, and other manifestations of having a body, specifically a female one. Against this ignorance and shame, the group deployed a process of collective learning and talking, acquiring knowledge and sharing experiences, emotions, and ideas: "The process of talking was as crucial as the facts themselves" (Boston Women's Health Book Collective 1973). This process became a model for feminist self-organization and arguably for a great many other social innovations in the following decades.

The book was highly influential, but not everything has changed. The experience of not being listened to, not being taken seriously, not being sufficiently informed, not daring to ask or not getting answers to one's questions is certainly still common in the medical context. There is still a general sense that the field of medicine, from medical practice via medical research to the politics of health and biomedicine, is a domain where experts reign supreme, exercising a paternalist type of rule, claiming to know what is best for the patient or the public, telling them what to do and what not to do, and making decisions while scarcely consulting with the persons concerned. Medical institutions are still widely experienced as a realm of heteronomy and alienation, a realm where people have to struggle in order to understand what is happening to them. People still often feel they are not allowed to express their wishes and fears, make themselves heard, and engage experts in dialogue rather than passively await their decisions. Self-determination, patient autonomy, participation and dialogue are still the watchwords of the struggle against medical domination.

At the same time, we have seen an explosion of discourse in relation to just about all practices and processes that in the 1970s were a matter of ignorance and shame, such as menstruation, masturbation, pregnancy, abortion, and death. These have now been joined by infertility, breast cancer, HIV, transgender, lesbian motherhood, reproductive technologies. Today, it has become an established norm that patients have to be informed, and that citizens need to be medically educated, if not genetically literate. Life has become a series of occasions for decisions that, as nearly everyone would agree, should *not* be taken by medical experts, but by the individual subject. We as individual subjects should decide whether, where, when and how we want to give birth, undergo breast cancer screening, cervical cancer vaccination, or genetic testing, which pregnancy we wish to abort and which we want to carry to term, which organs we want to donate, and even when, where and how (although not whether) we want to die. While people still experience medical paternalism, paternalism has become a pejorative term and self-determination a legitimate claim.

In 2007, an article in the Journal of Health Services Research & Policy hailed the changes incited by Our Bodies, Ourselves:

> The Collective, along with other self-help health and consumer groups that emerged in the late 1960s, played a critical role in transforming patients from passive recipients of health care into active consumers. Today's concept of shared decision-making in health care is firmly rooted in the principles and practices of health communication set forth in Our Bodies, Ourselves. Scholars now debate which patients prefer being active decision-makers and even ask if passive patients should be urged to take more active roles in decision-making. These controversies reflect the diffusion of models of doctor-patient communication and relationships that the book set out to create over three decades ago. (Ruzek 2007: 182)

In short, the norm of "the doctor knows best" has been replaced by the norm of shared decision-making, the figure of the ignorant and docile patient by the informed and active consumer, and the commandment to keep silent by the commandment to talk. Yet, if we are supposed to talk, what is to be our language? If we are supposed be informed consumers, what menu are we supposed to choose from? And if we are supposed to make decisions, what if we do not want to decide? If communication takes us on the road to liberation, what are the terms on which communication takes place? And what is the meaning of the liberation we are thereby offered?

If we take a second look at Our Bodies, Ourselves of 1970, we find that some things apparently got lost in transformation. The kind of liberation the group had in mind did *not* equate to consumer choice, shared decision-making, and health communication. Their ideas had something to do with social and political change and social justice, and not just with models of communication:

The factors in our society which produce a great amount of sickness are not dealt with by the medical establishment. In fact, bad housing, poor nutrition, poor sanitation, pollution, and dangerous working conditions are not dealt with by any establishment. The diseases resulting from these factors are obviously suffered mainly by poor people who have no control over them. (Boston Women's Health Collective 1970: 179)

The idea that one has to have control in order to be liberated has endured, but it has been detached from the political meaning it carried in the movement context at the time. Having control is certainly important today, particularly in the medical context, but the struggle for control, so the common understanding, is the struggle against doctors who prescribe medication without explaining it properly or who refuse to accept your living will; it is not the struggle against poverty, dangerous working conditions, or pollution. Today, to speak of bad housing or poor sanitation in relation to liberation would sound somewhat outmoded. Some readers would intuitively respond that these social problems have been solved or at least dramatically mitigated. However, this is unfortunately not the case—or, at the very least, it depends where you look. Similarly, to speak of power, class, race, or the profits made in the health sector, like the Boston women's group did, would seem rather inappropriate for today's active consumer.

William Arney and Bernard Bergen (1984) have provided us with a different view on the changes in modern medicine since the 1950s. They also register the entrance of the speaking subject into the medical setting, that is, the patient speaking about her- or himself, and thereby contributing to the therapeutic process rather than obstructing it. Arney and Bergen describe the new vision of patients as partners or participants, as proclaimed by medical textbooks in the 1950s and 1960s. However, they refuse to celebrate these changes as marking a transition from oppression to liberation, from medical domination to self-determination, from depersonalized medical care to the humane recognition of the person, or from authoritarian to egalitarian relations. Drawing on Foucault's critique of the repression hypothesis and his insight that speaking the truth about oneself is not an act against power but within power, they insist that "the person does not dissolve the activity of power as he or she begins to speak" (Arney and Bergen 1984: 5). Power is not just domination and exclusion; today it also works through *in*clusion. Thus, Arney and Bergen argue that "[w]e may have to suspend the seemingly self-evident idea that to study power we must focus on exclusionary practices" (Arney and Bergen 1984: 6). This view generates a new set of questions. If we are invited to participate, in what do we participate? On whose terms, in which terms, in which setting, within which framework? If we are invited to talk, in which language? If we are supposed to take decisions by ourselves, what does it mean to decide? And what does it mean to render things decidable at all?

Today, we maintain, the changes pointed out by Arney and Bergen go beyond the scope of the medical encounter. The contributions to this volume show how the incitement to talk, the invitation to speak about oneself, to search for, to express and to share one's preferences, anxieties, views and values has been cultivated in different settings and incorporated into a wide range of practices and institutions, from labor wards to living wills, from counseling services, ethics committees and public participation arrangements, to regulation processes or policy debates. Today, in many settings, not only patients talk about themselves, but also professionals, citizens, and at times even experts and policy-makers. They all are constructed as partners in communicative procedures that require them to participate by means of speaking about themselves. If Foucault traces the speaking subject from the confessional to psychotherapy, and Arney and Bergen follow her from there to the medical encounter, today we also find her in the consulting room, the ethics committee, in public consultations, and parliamentary debates—or at home discussing with her children how to fill in the form of her living will. Part of this development may be understood as a consequence of the transformations described by Arney and Bergen, namely that medicine transcends the boundaries of the doctor-patient dyad by taking over, or being charged with, novel responsibilities from managing chronic disease, via prevention or containing health care costs, to recruiting medical subjects or procuring organs for transplant. Medicine takes on the logic of systems, turning both doctor and patient, along with other professionals such as midwives, nurses, counselors, or pastors, into team members and participants in systemic processes. Team members, to some extent, have to speak a common language, but what language is it? What can and what cannot be said in this "proper talk" (Braun/Moore/Herrmann/Könninger 2010)?

The systemic turn in medicine is not the only strand that has led to the proliferation of practices of speaking-about-oneself. Another strand goes back to the new social movements of the 1970s and 1980s, such as the feminist, gay, disability rights, or the environmental movements, which questioned expert authority, demanded self-determination, institutional transparency, citizen participation, and attention to the value dimension of policy-making. Interestingly, many institutional innovations that incorporate the speaking subject, such as non-directive counseling, shared decision-making in peer committees, or public consultations on contested policy issues, have evolved in issue areas for which medicine claims competency, such as dying or withdrawal of treatment (see the contributions by Isabella Jordan and Helen Kohlen in this volume), giving birth or being pregnant (see the contributions by Marion Schumann and Silja Samerski), political controversies on genetic technology and reproductive medicine or other contentious medical technologies in the political arena (see the contributions by Svea L. Herrmann, Sabine Könninger, and Kathrin Braun and Susanne Schultz), or contraception and population policy in the context of development policy (see the contribution by Susanne Schultz).

If this observation is correct, it may have to do with the fact that the body is still at the intersection between the personal and the political, at the point where processes of subjectivation and processes of government meet. On the one hand, we experience our body as the most personal thing to us. Decisions about our body, we feel, should be a matter of personal autonomy and not of doctors, experts or policy-makers' authority. This is the more so when it comes to moments in life we experience as deeply personal and often difficult, such as being pregnant, giving birth, trying to conceive a child, or facing death. On the other hand, the body and the "facts of life", such as health and disease, fertility and infertility, conceiving or not conceiving a child, aging and dying, are located where Foucault saw sexuality, namely at the intersection between the individual and the population, the techniques of discipline and the mechanisms of regulation, anatomo-politics and biopolitics (Foucault 2002: 250f.). For politics today, matters of health and illness, reproduction and mortality are no less important than for classical biopolitics in the 19th and early 20th century, for they are still linked to matters of economic productivity, social welfare, public finances, or political conflict, and as such they are in need of government and steering. For these reasons, as Foucault has shown, medicine has been critical for articulating the formation of governmental technologies, knowledge and subjectivities, from the emergence of the modern state up to the present. In contrast to the era of classical biopolitics, however, social engineering is no longer considered a legitimate technology for governing the living, as it had been in the first half of the 20th century. In the first part of the 20th century, one could say, two historic novelties, which Foucault inspected in The Will to Knowledge (Foucault 1980), still existed largely in separation from each other, namely the migration of confession practices into the therapeutic setting and the emergence of a novel type of power regulating, managing and enhancing the life processes of the population. Foucault dealt with these two phenomena in separate chapters. True, they were articulated through sexuality, forming the link between the individual and the reproduction of the population as well as the site of knowledge production, truth telling, categorization and normalization. Yet they occurred in different institutional contexts and on different social levels. Confession practices, soul searching and subjectivation took place on the micro level and mainly in the context of psychotherapy, whereas this new type of power Foucault named biopower was located at the macro level, exercised by state actors through public policies, and supported by experts, professionals, charities and other intermediaries. The appearance of the speaking person, with her respective practices of soul searching and subjectivation, was confined to the micro level, and even here more specifically to dyadic settings that still bore some resemblance to the penitent-priest relation. Even the ordinary medical encounter between doctor and patient, as Arney and Bergen showed, gave no appropriate environment for the person speaking about herself. Way into the 1950s, it did not give rise to self-technologies in form of introspection and truth telling. Looking, not listening, was the usual way of finding out what was wrong. The doctor was the one, who had the relevant knowledge to interpret the signs of disease on, or in, the patient's body, the patient had to show those signs and follow instructions, and ideally disease would go away. Likewise, at the level of biopolitics, the population, in its size, composition, health, birth rate, death rate, productivity, proclivity to alcoholism, crime, or other deviant behavior, was the target of governing and steering, exercised top down, through the application of expert knowledge, transformed into provisions and measures to be followed (ideally) by the target groups, such that social problems would go away. In the 20th century, biopolitics has largely taken the form of social engineering in this sense: identifying a "social problem", making a decision upon the means of intervention, applying appropriate expert knowledge, implementing schemes and programs—everything in a top down manner, and ideally solving the social problem. Within this model there was no room, nor need, for speaking subjects. Medical knowledge and medical professionals have been prominently involved in this type of biopolitical social engineering, designing and implementing policy schemes for hygiene, eugenics, and so on. In short, while the speaking subject made its appearance in the therapeutic setting on the micro level, medicine and biopolitics for decades remained a paternalist, expert-led, top down affair. Technologies of the self were linked to but not integrated with technologies of government.

The contributions to this volume suggest that since the 1960s, and in a variety of fields, we have seen the mutual assimilation and integration of self-technologies and governmental technologies. In the course of this integration, the figure of the speaking person has hugely expanded her range of activities, moving from the narrow, dyadic, therapeutic setting, via the medical encounter, the clinic, or the ethics board, further into the political realm. Self-examination, self-expression, and self-determination have become widely accepted norms and values both in relation to an increasing range of issues of "delegated biopolitics" (Memmi 2003), such as abortion, preimplantation genetic diagnosis, embryo research, or medically assisted suicide, and in relation to a plethora of arenas and institutional settings. The range of arenas where it is considered acceptable, and even virtuous, to examine one's feelings, to express them as authentically as possible, and to make decisions on the basis of them has expanded greatly compared with the 1950s and 1960s. However, the studies assembled in this volume also show that when claims to self-expression and self-determination are incorporated into new institutional contexts, this has certain implications, such as the requirement to use a certain language that allows for addressing some things but not others, the requirement to accept certain terms of participation upon entering the communication (for instance about which issue is at stake and which is not), and to accept certain new norms and standards that have replaced older ones. New types of expectations and necessities emerge, like the expectation that one plans ahead for one's death or calculates whether or not to abort a fetus on the basis of statistical probabilities. We know from the growing body of governmentality studies, that the self is increasingly engaged in new technologies of government, particularly through new choices, new freedoms but also new responsibilities brought about by technoscientific developments in genetics, reproductive medicine, neuroscience, pharmacology and other medical fields (Lemke 2004; Rose 2007). The studies presented here add to this field. However, the focus of this book is not specifically on the production of a neoliberal subjectivity in and through techno-scientific advancements. It focuses on forms of interaction rather than individualization, and on changing social practices rather than techno-scientific developments and their implications. Many of the changes examined here, such as the invention of ethics committees or living wills, were *not* induced by technoscientific developments, although public discourse gives the impression that they were. We do not intend to sustain this belief, for to do so would mean, even if unwillingly, subscribing to technological determinism.

Also, our interest is very much on the dark sides of these transformations, on what gets lost and what cannot be said and done, and on the new burdens, norms, demands and impositions that emerge. We think something else is going on in relation to medicine and biopolitics besides the responsibilization of the individual, although this is an important part of the story. We think that new forms of interaction have evolved that to some extent incorporate the notion of self-determination and participation and that operate as new social technologies for managing different types of conflicts and crises. These are social technologies that, unlike technologies of classical social engineering, cannot operate *without* the speaking person being actively involved. Also, unlike medical or expert paternalism, they do not consist of telling people what they must and must not do. These new social technologies are procedural rather than prescriptive and directive. What does that mean, and what is the difference? In order to understand what is new, it may be useful to compare the concept of social engineering to the concept of procedure.

In The Open Society and its Enemies, first published in 1944, Karl Popper conceptually differentiates piecemeal social engineering and utopian social engineering, defending the former against the latter. For Marx, he argues, capitalism subjects everyone, workers and capitalists alike, to its immanent laws. Capitalism is a machinery that works blindly and makes everybody blind (Popper 2003: 123f.). Therefore, Popper argues, according to Marx, there can be no way of rationally improving the system: "Social engineering is impossible, and a social technology therefore useless" (Popper 2003: 124). People will not be better off until the system has been replaced by a better one. Piecemeal social engineering, in contrast, is more realistic, less problematic, and, in Popper's view, definitely possible. It seeks to fight the greatest social evils through rational, science-based political interventions such as tax systems, social insurances, police forces, educational systems and the like. Piecemeal social engineering basically means rational planning, exercised by governments, informed by social science, and applied to social institutions. It presupposes a clear, substantial idea of the problems at stake and what needs to be changed.

In the 1960s, the term social engineering became linked to a growing discourse on "social problems", mainly in the US. Social problems could be anything from war and poverty to pollution, traffic, alcoholism or the growth of the "world population". Within this discourse, the "social engineer" does not tackle institutions, such as tax or social insurance systems as in Popper, so much as individual behavior. Social problems, within this discourse, are caused by inappropriate human behavior and the key to solving them is to alter human behavior. The job of the social engineer is to bring people, for instance, "to have fewer babies, or to drive more carefully or to refrain from disliking blacks" (Weinberg 1991: 42). Thus, it presupposes the idea of governments as coherent subjects who have both the capacity and the right to identify social problems, set policy goals, and use top-down interventions to achieve them. Above all, it implies the idea that governments are entitled to set substantial policy goals. At each stage of this process, they are to be supported by reliable, readily applicable social science knowledge that allows for rational planning.

Yet, almost at the same historic moment when the idea of social engineering becomes popularized, it also becomes problematized. Questions arise whether social engineering, with its substantial goals and its centralized schemes, is compatible with individual freedom. What are its costs, and does it work at all? It turns into a polemic concept mobilized by those who fear for their financial resources or their liberties or both, endangered by patronizing governments. Now "social engineering" has become a pejorative term. It has taken on the meaning of illegitimate and expansive government intervention. Certainly the classic model of social engineering has not disappeared completely. In those parts of the Western world, however, that subscribe to advanced liberal strategies of government, which have been on the rise since the 1980s, it has largely been replaced by ideas of "government at a distance" (Rose and Miller 1992). We think that in these contexts, governing through procedure has become an important technology of governing at a distance across different social realms and levels. Although the concept of procedure may have a technicist or bureaucratic, impersonal ring to it, the speaking subject is in fact at the center of governing through procedure. In order to understand this concept, it is useful to turn to a sociologist who has described the functional logic of procedures, even if in a different context than ours, namely Niklas Luhmann. In his *Legitimation durch Verfahren*, first published in 1969, Luhmann (1983) analyzes what kind of legitimacy is created through modern decision-making processes by courts, parliaments and public administrations, and *how* it is created. He argues that in these processes legitimacy is derived specifically from the organization of decision-making as procedure. One does not have to subscribe to the view of social theory as systems theory in order to make use of this analysis. While Jürgen Habermas has accused Luhmann's systems theory of *operating as* a social technology, we think his concept of procedure can be useful in order to *analyze* a new type of social technology. Luhmann, Habermas argues, excludes questions of practical reasoning, that is normative questions, from his conceptualization of the social order (Habermas and Luhmann 1985). In doing so, Habermas says, Luhmann reframes practical questions as technical questions and depoliticizes them, thereby protecting the existing social order from being challenged in public discourse. However, sometimes refraining from taking a normative stance can actually be quite useful for developing a critical stance, as Foucault (who has been the target of a similar critique by Habermas) has shown.

Now, what is a procedure? In order to understand the specificity of procedure, one may start with what a procedure is not. For instance, a procedure is not a rule or a set of rules. Although procedures are mostly regulated by a legal framework, they are not identical with it. Rules exist; they may be formal or informal, be enforced or suspended, applied or ignored. Procedures take place. Their form of existence is a temporal one; they can only exist as practices in time. Further, procedures are not rituals. Oftentimes, procedures may have strong ritual elements, but this is not what makes them procedures. A ritual is a fixed sequence of actions within which only one action is correct at a time; there is no choice among different equally possible options. In a procedure, by contrast, the outcome is uncertain. If it is not, it is a ritual and not a procedure. It is the uncertainty of the outcome and the existence of choices that motivates people to participate in a procedure at all; if the outcome was clear, there would be no point in participating.

In *Legitimation durch Verfahren*, Luhmann looks at legislative procedures, court trials, and bureaucratic procedures, that is, those procedures that in modern societies generate, interpret or implement the law. His aim is to reconstruct the problem to which these procedures are the solution. Note, that the question is not which particular problems are solved within particular procedures, but rather which problems are solved through procedure as such. In the case of the above mentioned type of procedures, namely those that generate, interpret or implement the law, the problem is to generate the legitimacy of the law under conditions of modern uncertainty, where legitimacy means the general willingness of people to accept, within certain limits of tolerance, the law as binding, regardless of whether it benefits their interests or is in line with their values or convictions, or not. Thus, legitimacy is not synonymous with consensus; the problem is how to secure legitimacy under conditions where consensus is unlikely. Due to the disappearance of natural law and its constraints, but also, one could add, to the growth of new options opened up through technoscientific developments, the range of possible alternative courses of action has greatly increased. Procedures are forms of interaction that, following Luhmann, serve to render things *decidable* and absorb the frustration and potential anger of those whose view did not prevail. They eliminate alternatives, neutralize energies, and dampen conflicts (Luhmann 1983: 4).

The point, thus, is not to create consensus, or to make the *right* decision, nor even to make *good* decisions. Procedures as such are not about the quality of the outcome, since there is rarely an uncontested way to assess outcome; they are about manageability. Procedures can be understood as social technologies for dealing with matters of uncertainty, conflict, or crisis in a way that avoids disruption, absorbs disturbances and allows for things to smoothly go on. This is not to say, however, that procedures always function the way they should and achieve what they are supposed to achieve, nor that without them, we would necessarily see an eruption of open protest. But it may explain why we see all sorts of procedures emerging in different contexts, some for decision-making, some just for deliberation, consideration, evaluation, argumentation or other speaking practices, even if people are not necessarily convinced that this leads to better outcomes, or any outcomes for that matter, let alone to a more efficient way of achieving those outcomes. Procedures serve to achieve manageability, not particular outcomes. But how do they achieve manageability? Referring to collective decision-making procedures, Luhmann argues that they consist of building a decision-history within which each single step turns into a fact that as such narrows the scope of possible subsequent steps. The UK Human Fertilisation and Embryology Authority, for instance, has a tool called a "decision tree". There are decision trees for different sorts of questions, for instance a "PGD decision tree" (HFEA 2010), or a decision tree for clinic staff (HFEA 2009). They all provide a scheme of "ifs" and "thens" that are meant to provide guidance for decision-making on different sorts of issues. While the decision tree is a highly standardized, computer program-like procedure, it is important to note that it is *not* a computer program. Decision-making is not left to software. These schemes, on the contrary, are tools for clinic staff (for instance) to organize their interaction with patients, or for members of the licensing committee to make a collective decision on whether or not to grant a clinic a license to perform preimplantation genetic diagnosis (PGD). A decision tree is a technology of interaction, not an electronic technology. Its purpose is not only to generate a decision—for that could be done by a computer program—but also to render issues decidable in a way that both clinic staff and patient, both license committee members and clinic, and in case of the latter, maybe even the general public, will feel committed to—even if they don't necessarily like the outcome.

Speaking is key to generating this commitment. The properly operating procedure will provide the patient, the staff, the committee member, and sometimes also the member of the public with an opportunity to speak. Through expressing herself, her thoughts, opinions, sometimes her beliefs, values or feelings, she participates in narrowing down the scope of possible future actions. Her utterances become part of the decision-making history, and they enter that history as facts she cannot easily undo. If she wants to be taken seriously, she needs to be credible and authentic, which means she has to be true to what she said before. If she missed the right moment for uttering protest, she cannot make good for it later; belated protest rings hollow and is easy to rebut (Luhmann 1983: 45).

Aside from binding participants to their utterances in the past, and thereby eliminating alternatives, Luhmann suggests that procedures also serve to fulfill expressive needs, such as letting out anger, or pride, or presenting oneself as a good, moral person. Thus, while the expected outcomes may lie in the distant future, the opportunity to speak may fulfill more immediate needs (Luhmann 1983: 124).

What happens is that upon entering into a procedure, the person accepts the terms on which the procedure takes place. To become a participant is to accept its rules, its setting, its remit and the like. Second, upon participating, the person binds herself to the history of her own expressions, to what she has or has not said at a certain moment in time. One effect is that for her it becomes hard to sustain fundamental opposition to the terms of the debate once she has subscribed to them. Another effect is that if she does not agree to the outcome but still sustains an attitude of opposition, conflict or anger, it is easy for society to ignore her. If she does not adjust to the new situation, she will just be the notorious grumbler.

Not all of the procedures examined in this volume are decision-making procedures, and few are as standardized as the "decision tree". We think there is a wide variety of procedures that serve as social technologies for rendering issues manageable, some more rule-based, some more informal, some more standardized, others more flexible, some restricted to a dyadic setting, such as genetic counseling, some to a restricted group of peers, such as ethics committees, some open to a diffuse public, such as public bioethics debates. What they have in common is that they make it hard for participants and non-participants to sustain conflict and opposition. For non-participants, the fact that mechanisms and procedures of ethical debate, shared decision-making, exploration of preferences and so on are in place, means that they *could* participate, if only they seriously wished to, or that, when the moment comes, they *will* be asked for informed consent, or that their case *will* be brought to the respective ethics committee. So, we can be reassured that there are proper procedures in place to take care of crisis when it occurs. Whether this is the type of care we actually need or wish for ourselves and those we love is another question, and one that becomes much harder to address once the proper procedures are in place. Being the active consumer, you can opt not to buy certain prenatal tests, but it is much harder to say that society does not need this type of test at all. You can get a lot of support from churches, charities, or call centers to fill out your living will, but you cannot wish just to give yourself into the hands of people you trust when you die. You can actively participate in public bioethics debates but if in this context you insist on talking about poverty, power, capitalism, or unequal health care you will most likely be told not to change the subject. This is not to say that self-determination, shared decision-making, participation, or ethical debate are *just* social technologies, and certainly not that they are novel, more insidious means of manipulation. Yet, we think, someone has to be the killjoy and question whether they really give so much cause for celebration, detached as they are from the struggle for political and social change.

The contributions to this volume pose this question, each on the basis of detailed empirical research in their field. In the first contribution, Marion Schumann has traced the emergence of the speaking person in the labor ward back into the 1950s. Using contemporary archive material, medical journals and books, as well as sources from the German women's magazine *Constanze,* she examines the transformation of obstetrical concepts in the Federal Republic of Germany between 1950 and 1975. Beginning with the traditional model of midwives assisting women giving birth at home, a practice that was still widespread in the early 1950s, she analyzes two scientific methods of childbirth that have been established in the clinic at different paces: technologically monitored and preventively calculated "programmed childbirth," and the so-called gentle, or "natural" childbirth model of Dick-Read. What emerges from this study is the "internal" connections between these two models, in that both show the predominance of thinking in terms of planning in the 1960s.

Isabella Jordan examines the transformations in dealing with death since the 1960s. Since then, she argues, the dying have increasingly been professionally cared for by clinical institutions. Developments in intensive care have raised the possibility of extending lives. The public debates in Germany since the 1970s on "euthanasia" on the one hand and on terminal care on the other both focus on "self-determination in the final phase of life" and the question of how it could best be achieved. They evoke peoples' alleged "fear of high-tech medicine" as well as their alleged demand for self-determination, suggesting the latter be the best solution to the former, in order to avoid "sustaining life at all costs." Based on document analysis, the contribution examines the development of the death debate in Germany. It traces how what were initially contrary demands for "euthanasia" on the one hand and terminal care on the other have in recent years converged in the demand for living wills. It shows that while the demand to plan or arrange one's own death is becoming more pronounced in public debates, everyday social and caregiving aspects based on responsibility and trust are being thematized less and less.

Silja Samerski investigates the concept of individual self-determination more closely in the context of genetic counseling. Based on an empirical study of genetic counseling in Germany, this contribution frames counseling for "self-determination" and "autonomy" as a new technique of social engineering. She argues that in the 20th century self-determination was a major goal for female activists struggling against cooptation of female fertility by the state, whereas today, counseling services in medicine impose "autonomous decisions" upon patients. Taking the example of prenatal genetic counseling, she shows that professionally taught self-determination creates several paradoxes. First, it is service dependent. The act of deciding is identified with selecting from a menu of service options. Second, it is mediated by technoscience. Clients are supposed to choose technical procedures, mostly ultrasound or amniocentesis, and base their decision on scientific constructs such as chromosome numbers and probability curves. Third, it is compulsory to choose because even rejection of the whole procedure will be interpreted as a choice, namely, for the no-test option with its associated risks. Therefore, this new kind of self-determination requires services offered by professionals, schooling in technoscience, and decision making between risk-laden options.

Helen Kohlen's contribution looks into shared decision-making and shifting responsibilities in hospital ethics committees. She shows how bedside ethics gave way to bioethics and how institutionalized committees have played a decisive role in this transformation process. The key questions here are: What makes people call upon experts of bioethics in hospital committees, and what are the consequences of collective decision-making and a rationalistic framework for resolving "patients' cases"? Bioethics, understood as a contested discipline and practice whose historical traces and proper tasks are not at all clear, has nonetheless grown rapidly as an interdisciplinary enterprise in the US since the 1960s, when bioethicists were called upon to serve as expert consultants in numerous medical, legal, political, educational, and industrial areas. In the 1970s, the "Case of Karen Quinlan" drove the idea of decision-making by local committees forward. Gradually bioethics moved into the medical field while ethics committees became the standard organizational form for discussions on patient care review and engagement in a collective decision-making process, the formulation of new rules and policies and the education of health care professionals on how to cope with ethical dilemmas. Medical morality gave way to bioethics by adopting not only its interdisciplinary approach, but also its rational analytical style and a technical procedure of principle-based ethics. The responsibility that once belonged to the authority of the medical profession, rooted in the Hippocratic oath, has shifted into a collective process of decision-making by a team of (bio-)ethics experts, physicians, lawyers, nurses, chaplains and social workers.

Moving to the arena of public debate, Svea Herrmann analyzes the political conflicts on embryonic stem cell research in the UK and in Germany in the late 1990s. She argues that public ethical debate, here, worked like a kind of "speaking cure for conflicts", arguing that problematization in terms of ethics underpinned a constant call for the stimulation of public discourse and the invitation of more and more participants in it. At the same time, these ethical debates did not counter a preexisting commitment to scientific "progress." On the contrary, in both countries, public discourse, especially a discourse in terms of ethics, was a medium in which an imperative of scientific progress, on the one hand, as well as actual or possible concerns or opposition towards scientific endeavor, on the other, could coexist. Ethical problematizations of these issues created a discursive space for the articulation of anxiety or conflicts and the formation of an ethical viewpoint, without, however, challenging an imperative of scientific progress. In face of new research options public participation in ethical debate was directed at the formation of a personal ethical perspective or at personal decision-making according to individual moral conviction rather than at political contestation of scientific progress. Thus, public ethical debates followed and worked in favor of liberal and individualistic market logic.

Kathrin Braun and Susanne Schultz also examine science policy controversies. They focus on the government of preimplantation genetic diagnosis (PGD) in the UK and argue that the mode of government that has emerged here differs from classical modernist statecraft in many crucial respects. It is a pragmatic, flexible, procedural mode of governance, which ranges from counseling processes among patients, clinics and the regulating authority, the Human Fertilisation and Embryology Authority (HFEA), via deliberation processes within the HFEA, to processes of debate organized through public consultations. This new mode of government, the authors argue, is characterized by incremental decision-making rather than by general rules, elastic and temporary categories rather than fixed ones, non-parliamentary bodies rather than parliament, and an emphasis on personal experiences, values, and emotions rather than universal principles. In effect, however, it is permissive and open to a gradual expansion of technoscientific practices. It does not per se give more room to political contestations, since it maintains an overall non-antagonistic constellation. Acknowledging uncertainty and incorporating extrascientific actors as well as extrascientific forms of knowledge are compatible with a permissive, pro technoscience stance.

Sabine Könninger also examines the social technologies of bioethics, but on the level of technoscience policy. Since the 1980s, she shows, we see the emergence and proliferation of ethics procedures and institutions, such as national ethics councils, in scientific governance in Western countries, mainly in the field of biotechnology. Although it seems self-evident that issues in biotechnology and medicine are ethical issues and that ethics bodies are therefore necessary, the discourse on nanotechnology shows that there is a process that goes beyond the linking of ethics and biotechnology: Not only the number of publicly sponsored procedures and bodies increases, but also the number of issues. Thus, we see a "new" proliferation of ethicpolitics. Based on an analysis of key documents, expert interviews and participant observations, the chapter examines the development and meaning of ethicpolitics in France, tracing back bio- and nanoethics discourses by identifying the shifts, differences and parallels in the ways they were problematized. On the example of the French National Ethics Committee, Könninger shows that nanotechnology became an ethical issue through being framed as a health issue and as an individual problem. Second, she argues that ethicpolitics is flexible in that it frames the way the discourse is performed, rather than providing substantive normative orientation for action or the shaping of bio- or nanotechnological developments.

Moving from the level of national public policy to international politics, Susanne Schultz investigates the articulation of demographic aims and gender policies in international population programs. She questions the claim that we live in an age of a "new biopolitics," marked predominantly by a regime of individualized self-responsibility and biological citizenship. This, she argues, is a one-sided view that overlooks the continuity of "old biopolitics," characterized by state-led and coercive practices and a focus on the administration of populations, outside the Western industrialized countries. It is true, she argues, that since the United Nations' Conference on Population and Development in Cairo 1994, the figure of the docile, receptive addressee of international population control policies has been replaced by the figure of the autonomous woman in the developing world who claims and responsibly manages her own "reproductive health". While such a shift towards self-determination, empowerment and women's reproductive autonomy, *has* taken place, Schultz shows, it operates not as the antithesis but rather as the new vehicle of a neo-Malthusian demographic rationality that seeks to reduce the number of the poor in the non-Western World. The new individualizing concepts, she shows, are articulated with demographic goals through an anti-natalist bias.

The editor and the authors of this volume wish to thank Alfred Moore for helpful comments and linguistic improvement, Andreas Sturm for reliable technical support, and Barbara Duden for long-standing inspiring discussions.

REFERENCES

Arney, William Ray/Bergen, Bernard Jay (1984): Medicine and the management of living. Taming the last great beast, Chicago and London: The University of Chicago Press.

Boston Women's Health Collective (1970): Women and their bodies. A course; available at http://www.ourbodiesourselves.org/uploads/pdf/OBOS1970.pdf (last accessed 12/10/2010).

Boston Women's Health Book Collective (1973): Preface from the 1973 edition of Our bodies, ourselves; available at http://www.ourbodiesourselves.org/about/1973obos.asp (last accessed 12/10/2010).

Braun, Kathrin/Moore, Alfred/Herrmann, Svea L./Könninger, Sabine (2010): "Governmental bioethics between the technological model and reflexive government", in: Economy & Society 39(4): pp. 510 - 533.

Foucault, Michel (1980): The history of sexuality. Vol. I: An introduction, New York: Vintage Books.

— (2002): Society must be defended. Lectures at the College de France 1975-1976, New York: Picador.

Habermas, Jürgen/Luhmann, Niklas (1985): Theorie der Gesellschaft oder Sozialtechnologie, Frankfurt a.M.: Suhrkamp.

HFEA (2009): Guidance supplement to Chair's Letter CH(10)05 and amended Directions 0005 and 0007; available at http://212.49.193.187/docs/Consent_options_for_releasing_patient_identifying_information.pdf (last accessed 12/21/2010).
— (2010): HFEA Licence Committee Meeting, 26 August 2010; available at http://guide.hfea.gov.uk/guide/ShowPDF.aspx?ID=4249 (last accessed 11/26/2010).
Lemke, Thomas (2004): "Disposition and determinism—genetic diagnostics in risk society", in: The Sociological Review 52(4), pp. 550-566.
Luhmann, Niklas (1983): Legitimation durch Verfahren, Frankfurt a.M.: Suhrkamp.
Memmi, Dominique (2003). "Governing through speech: The new state administration of bodies", in: Social Research 70(2), pp. 645-658.
Popper, Karl (2003): The open society and its enemies. Volume two: Hegel and Marx, New York: Routledge.
Rose, Nikolas (2007): The politics of life itself. Biomedicine, power, subjectivity in the twenty-first century, Princeton: Princeton University Press.
Ruzek, Sheryl (2007): "Transforming doctor-patient relationships", in: Journal of Health Services Research & Policy 12(3), pp. 181-181.
Weinberg, Alvin M. (1991): "Can technology replace social engineering?" in: William B. Thompson (ed), Controlling technology: contemporary issues, Buffalo, N.Y.: Prometheus Books, pp. 41-48.

From social care to planning childbirth in the Federal Republic of Germany 1950-1975

MARION SCHUMANN

In the first half of the 20th century, childbirth in Germany was still considered a fateful event. It primarily took place in the social environment of the pregnant woman's home with the assistance of a midwife and only required medical aid in an emergency. By the mid-1970s, clinical childbirth had established itself in Germany nationwide. The scientification of assisting childbirth that accompanied hospitalization had converted childbirth into a procedure that could be planned and controlled. A thrust in the direction of planning and rationalization in obstetrics can be detected in particular in the 1960s, a time when new childbirth models were being developed. This was a decade in which German society was fixated on progress and predictability, and a previously unknown optimism expressed itself in the notion that the future could be shaped (Döring-Manteuffel 2000: 663; Schildt 2000: 21ff.). A planning culture also worked its way into assisting childbirth. While childbirth was essentially an incalculable event until well into the 1950s with an uncertain beginning, course, and outcome, with the advent of the scientification of assisting childbirth, a thinking in terms of planning and control moved into the delivery rooms. In the following, I will introduce the various childbirth concepts that were available during the period of investigation and present their planning orientation, drawing on my research into the history of midwifery in the Federal Republic, which is based on material from medical journals and books as well as popular magazines, in particular the women's magazine *Constanze* (Schumann 2009).[1]

ASSISTING CHILDBIRTH IN HOME MIDWIFERY

Until the mid-1950s, childbirth, which was assisted by a self-employed midwife, primarily took place in the home. In order to practice home midwifery as a self-employed midwife, she required official authorization in the form of permission to establish a business (HebG [Midwife Act] 1954: Section 10). At the same time, she was assigned a district in which to practice and was subject to direct control by the responsible public health officer. Midwives were authorized to practice their profession independently; a physician only had to be consulted if there were complications. In contrast, physicians were not allowed to oversee childbirth without enlisting a midwife. Midwives were awarded the monopoly on "normal" childbirth in 1938 by National Socialist law (HebG 1938: Section 3). Within this framework, the law required every pregnant woman to consult a midwife and hence made the midwife the all-embracing controlling authority for women giving birth at home (Lisner 2006: 99).[2] At the same time, the state controlled the midwives' practice of their profession and their private lives by way of public health officers, so that, as Wiebke Lisner shows, the National

---

1   The study was conducted within the scope of the DFG research focus "Professionalisierung, Organisation, Geschlecht" (Professionalization, Organization, Gender) and was funded as the subproject "Professionalisierung von Hebammen in Westdeutschland 1945-1975" (Professionalization of Midwives in West Germany 1945-1975).

2   The one-sided obligation did not, however, apply for the hospital, where if a physician was present the midwife was his subordinate (Section 43/2 of the Hebammendienstordnung [Official Midwife Regulations]). It was not until the Midwife Act was reformed in 1985, when home childbirth was again in demand in large cities, that gynecologists vehemently argued against the one-sided obligation. The law responded to women's explicit wish for female care only outside of the hospital through midwives and incorporated the one-sided obligation to enlist a midwife (see Schumann 2006).

Socialist state exercised dual control over midwives and women giving birth.

The home birth midwife independently and continuously supervised a woman, and later the newborn child as well, during pregnancy and childbirth, the postpartum period, and the first ten days of the newborn's life. She was often rooted in the milieu of her work district (ibid. 202ff.). This meant that she generally came from the same social environment as the pregnant woman, had for the most part spent her whole life in the same place, had had children herself there, and had only left her hometown during the period of her training. Midwives and their clients therefore not only had the same living environment, midwives moreover performed their job in the women's own homes. Thus, they had insight into the living conditions of the women and families they cared for, including into their sexuality, which the midwife's sphere directly impacted (ibid. 203). The law envisaged the unavoidable proximity between the midwife and her client to be a relationship marked by trust. On this point, Section 3 of the Midwife Act of 1938 (as well as that from 1954) states the following: "The Act has upheld the principle of the independent choice of a midwife in order that the pregnant woman enlist the midwife of her trust" (Zimdars/Sauer 1955: 23). In their description of their activity, midwives made special reference to this relationship with parturients, which they called a "relationship of trust" (Grabrucker 1996; Grubenmann 1993, 1995; Linner 1989). According to Lisner, for the NS state, the "special" meaning of midwifery lay in this relationship—it functionalized the closeness to women and their families and made midwives the connecting link between the health authority and families. Midwives had a dual mandate (Lisner 2006: 167f.). On the one hand, they were obligated to the state, and, on the other, to women. However, midwives and women giving birth were dependent on one another. The midwife counted on women being satisfied with her job, liking her personally, commissioning her, and not a colleague, to provide assistance. The women, on the other hand, relied on the discretion of the midwives, who gained insight into the various areas of their personal lives. According to Lisner, there was mutual social control in the supervision of home childbirth (ibid. 202ff.). During the pregnancy, birth, and postpartum recovery period, the midwife played a central role in the life of the woman she was attending to, for example as an adviser, listener, confidante, girlfriend, and for some women as a mother figure (ibid. 224). During the period of care, the relationship between the midwife and her client was intense, however, it eventually abated. The home birth midwife provided a service that she tailored to fit the individual parturient and her family. According to Lisner, she felt socially responsible for "her" women even beyond the scope of her midwifery tasks. Self-employed midwives in the Federal Republic also viewed their relationship to women as the core of their profession. The "personal aspect" was regarded as the midwife's strength, as reported in the *Hebammenzeitschrift* (Midwife Magazine) in the early 1950s (Schumann 2009: 85).

Beyond this, one of the goals of assisting childbirth was relieving labor pains, which obstetrics began advancing in the early 20th century by administering medication (Olbrich 1996: 6, 89). Physicians justified this by saying that it was desired by the women giving birth. As the biographical records of midwives show, home birth midwives, whom lawmakers never authorized to administer pain medication, often used a variety of different heat applications or massage in order to relieve labor pains (Grabrucker 1996; Grubenmann 1993, 1995; Linner 1989). They also attempted to bridge the period between contractions by distracting the women, for example by performing housework, doing needlework, playing cards, or going for a walk. Midwives saw a further form of support in their mere presence, talking to the women or simply holding their hand (Henze 1999: 58ff.). It often also happened that the women in labor "screamed bloody murder" and that the midwife was unable to comfort them. As a rule, however, she had a positive influence on the women, as Ricarda Henze (1999) learned from interviews with midwives.

The model of assisted childbirth at home ensured that women were accompanied by a midwife they were familiar with for the entire duration of the birth to whom they could address their needs and who, in the ideal case, could respond to these needs. The women had great freedom to move in their private sphere into which they, however, had to allow the midwives insight. Because the exact time of the birth could not be planned, both women had to flexible in terms of time, as the babies arrived when they arrived.

HOSPITALIZATION OF CHILDBIRTH

In 1954, half of all births in the Federal Republic took place in the home, the other half in the hospital. According to contemporary study results, above all young women, in particular those giving birth for the first time, preferred the hospital (Beske 1958: 158; Fitzek 1957: 6f., 23). These studies also show a clear connection between hospital childbirth and the social status of those giving birth, as the higher a level of education a woman had, the more likely she was to deliver her child in the hospital (Scherer 1970: 56). However, these differences blurred in the 1960s, and the hospital birth reached all classes, in particular those women giving birth for the first time. At that time, women regarded being attended to by a physician, or at least their spatial proximity, as the best condition for the birth of their child (Beske 1967: 453). The hospital was in general regarded as the place that promised security through the professional supervision of childbirth by medical experts. In addition, women were attracted by the pain relief medication that was available in the hospital (Declercq et al 2001: 25). Beyond this, health insurance paid for a ten-day postpartum hospital stay. Women in childbed thus had a period of recovery from the family and received instruction in the care of the newborn child.[3] For a mixture of these as well as further reasons, the share of hospital deliveries constantly rose: in 1960, already more than two thirds of all women gave birth to their children in hospital, and by 1970 this number had risen to 99 percent.[4] Despite the striking lack of staff and beds in hospitals (Simon 2000: 79ff.), which meant that women had to be cared for in makeshift beds or released on the third day after childbirth, according to the *Hebammenzeitschrift* (Schumann 2009: 62f.), they flocked to the hospitals, where they did not always receive care in line with the applicable standards. Thus, the ten-day postpartum recovery period was frequently cut short. Bottlenecks in the care of puerperas also existed in other industrial countries; here, however, they were cush-

---

3   There are no studies available on this subject. In the interviews I conducted with midwives, however, they time and again pointed out that many women regarded the period of postpartum recovery in the hospital as a luxury.
4   Hospital delivery rate: 1960: 66%, 1965: 83%, 1970: 95%. On the shift of the location where women gave birth and the conditions in the hospitals (see Schumann 2009, 54-66).

ioned by health policy. In Great Britain, doctors only allowed women who had just given birth be released early if it was guaranteed that they would be cared for by a midwife at home (Springborn 1964). At the same time, the health policy there attempted to avoid this situation by having births without complications first and foremost supervised by home birth care (Lindner 2004: 475). Such provisions were not allowed for in the Federal Republic, neither by health policymakers nor hospitals. Here, the hospitalization of childbirth was not planned and it was not accompanied by health policy measures, despite the lack of hospital beds that prevailed at the time.

FRAGMENTATION OF ASSISTING CHILDBIRTH AND MEDICALIZATION OF CHILDBIRTH

In hospitals, the assistance of childbirth was increasingly organized based on the division of labor. So-called attending midwives supervised a large share of the births in smaller hospitals until the late 1960s. They were not employed by the hospitals but worked freelance. They initially often accompanied women they knew to the clinic, tended to them during the entire childbirth process, sometimes for the duration of the postpartum recovery period, and in part cared for the newborn child. The sphere of activity of the attending midwives was gradually reduced to the delivery room, they increasingly worked in shifts like the midwives employed by hospitals, and with the end of the baby boom (Niehuss 2001: 376ff.) in Germany in the 1960s, the employed delivery room midwife predominated. She cared for women in the delivery room, worked in shifts, and the areas of postpartum recovery and newborn care were taken over by nurses. The assistance of childbirth in hospital based on the division of labor turned the activity of the midwife in the delivery room into a specialized working area oriented toward the physician, medicine, and technology. There was no provision for continuous one-on-one care by a midwife in hospital. The relationship between the midwife and the woman giving birth was anonymous and rationalized. While in 1938 a midwife assisted an average of 57 births a year, by 1955 this number had risen to 76, and in 1965 it was 129 (Schumann 2009: 71). The individual midwife supervised more and more births in hospital. In contrast to assisted childbirth in the home, the relationship between the midwife and the woman bearing the child was no longer characterized by mutual social dependence but by distance. Concurrent with the increasing share of hospital deliveries, until 1970, the profession of midwife gradually adapted to the generally accepted standards in the working world. Unlike the freelance midwife, the delivery room midwife had regular working hours, a secure income, and her personal life was separate from her professional life. While the midwife was still largely responsible for "normal" births in the delivery room, she was subordinate to the physician.

Obstetrics in hospitals in large cities experienced a further transformation in the 1950s due to the tendency to intervene in the course of childbirth. The principle of *nil nocere*, or skilled intervention, that marked classic obstetrics gradually lost relevance in the delivery room (Duden 1998: 161; Frasch 1987: 81), and an increase in Cesarean sections indicated a softening of the indication. Patience, an elementary requirement in traditional obstetrics, was increasingly abandoned (Goecke 1962: 22). In addition to the threefold increase in the rate of Cesarean sections in the 1950s, from one to three percent, other forms of intervention in childbirth became routine. This included administering anticonvulsant and analgesic medication. The administration of drugs to accelerate labor also rose significantly: in Munich's university clinic, the use of such drugs increased twofold between 1950 and 1960, which can only in part be explained by higher birth rates. In the same period, the number of episiotomies performed in this clinic went from virtually zero to 75 percent (Loytved 2004). In the opinion of the physicians, these interventions lessened the pain of childbirth and reduced the average duration of childbirth by two and a half hours, which in turn reduced the strain on the woman giving birth and her child. It was from this preventive point of view that doctors intervened in childbirth as soon as the respective means were available to the hospitals, as these interventions were believed to be harmless and not lead to complications.

The obstetrical practice by West German physicians in the 1950s tied in with the principles of assisting childbirth in the early 20th century. At the time, the opinion generally prevailed that labor pains, just like other painful states, were to be relieved with the aid of medication (Olbrich 1996: 8). There were various pharmacological agents available to doctors in the 1950s: these included groups of medication that could be administered orally, intravenously, intramuscularly, or rectally and which were in part subject to the German Narcotics Act. There was also laughing gas (nitrous oxide)—women in labor could activate the inhaler and thus control the narcosis themselves. This gas, which is still used today, led to a temporary interruption in consciousness and a sleep-like state. This also applies to the so-called passage narcoses that the doctor administers intravenously when he suspects the child's head will appear with the upcoming contraction (Martius/Gschwendter 1959: 113f.). The woman giving birth would soon fall asleep and the episiotomy performed without her being aware of it. She was not conscious during childbirth. However, the medication not only brought about the desired pain relief in the mother, as specialist literature reported, it also had a negative effect on the newborn's state of health via the placenta, especially if it was not dosed properly (ibid. 114f.). But the use of local anesthetics was also on the rise.[5]

It was primarily due to the use of anesthetic agents that the female readership of *Constanze,* at the time the most popular women's magazine with the highest circulation, began to criticize unconscious childbirth in the 1950s. It will be shown below that many of these women desired an alternative to this clinical practice, one of which they believed to be the "natural childbirth" propagated by the British gynecologist Grantly Dick-Read.

COUNTER-CONCEPT TO THE CLINIC: "NATURAL" CHILDBIRTH ACCORDING TO DICK-READ

The pioneer of the "psychologization" of obstetrics, the British physician Grantly Dick-Read (1890–1959), criticized the increasing intervention in childbirth in hospitals as early as the 1930s (Dick-Read 1960: 120ff.). In England, the share of hospital deliveries in the mid-1930s was 40 percent (Lisner 2006: 116).[6] In the 1920s, Read complained about the routine, indiscriminate administration by British doctors of anesthetics during childbirth in hospital (amnesic half-sleep, pain-free "alert childbirth"). In addition to other social influences, the administration of medication by gynecologists in the hospital, which was a matter of course, contributed to

---

5 In obstetrics, these included perineal infiltration as well as pudendal, caudal, sacral, and spinal anesthesia (see Martius/Gschwendter 1959, 87-96).
6 In Germany, in 1935 the delivery rate in clinics was 25%. Yet despite the promotion of the home birth system by the National Socialist state, by 1939 it had reached 39% (Lisner 2006: 100).

women expecting childbirth to be a primarily harrowing and painful event (Dick-Read 1960: 64ff.). A lack of positive role models for giving birth and the medical profession's focus on relieving labor pain had led to the development of "cultural labor,"[7] which he contrasted with "natural" childbirth.[8] The administration of medication had even resulted in fatalities. He furthermore attacked his professional counterparts: they forced women to take medication and did not respect their wishes (ibid. 1960: 118ff.). According to Read, the influences mentioned led to the pain of childbirth in the first place, which he considered to be a cultural phenomenon. In his opinion, childbirth was for the most part a painless occurrence:

Superstition, civilization and culture have brought influences to bear upon the minds of women which have introduced justifiable fears and anxieties concerning labor. The more cultured the races of the earth have become, so much the more positive have they been in pronouncing childbirth to be a painful and dangerous ordeal. Thus fear and anticipation have given rise to natural protective tensions in the body, and such tensions are not of the mind only, for the mechanism of protective action by the body includes muscle tension. Unfortunately, the natural tension produced by fear influences those muscles which close the womb and oppose the dilation of the birth canal during labor. Therefore, fear inhibits; that is to say, gives rise to resistance at the outlet of the womb, when in the normal state those muscles should be relaxed and free from tension. This resistance gives rise to pain, because the uterus is supplied with sensitive nerve endings which record pain arising from excessive tension. Therefore, Fear, Tension and Pain are three evils opposed to the natural design. (Dick-Read 2006: 38f.)

According to Read, tension was to be released and replaced by physical and emotional relaxation.

---

7   By cultural labor Read refers "to women who are physiologically and mechanically well-equipped but not prepared for childbirth. They have doubts and fears and they understand little of what is going on or the sensations they will be called upon to interpret correctly" (Dick-Read 2006: 271).
8   For Read, natural childbirth was "childbirth in which no physical, chemical or psychological condition is likely to disturb the normal sequence of events or disrupt the natural phenomena of parturition" (Dick-Read 2006: 269).

Thus, Read contrasted "natural" childbirth with "cultural labor." While he regarded the former as the norm, he viewed "cultural labor" as culturally modified and falsified. He did not believe childbirth to be either "an abnormal occurrence" or an illness, but saw it as "an achievement that resulted in the well-being of mothers and children" (Dick-Read 1978: 8), a "great physical effort" (ibid. 18). He assumed that a learning process would facilitate the reintroduction of the "natural" into obstetrics. He therefore developed a four-point program for women: the pregnant women was to become familiar with physical processes during pregnancy and childbirth and obtain information about proper nutrition during pregnancy. In his view, this contributed to "raising awareness about pregnancy and delivery" (Dick-Read 1960: 139). Point two concerned exercises for relaxing the body, which were meant to prevent tension during labor. Read called the third point tolerance exercises, which were intended to keep the pregnant woman's body flexible and prepare it for the effort that was to be demanded of it. The fourth point referred to breathing techniques, for according to Read, "controlled breathing" was very important for the great physical demand placed on women during childbirth in order to supply the muscles with a sufficient amount of oxygen. In addition, proper breathing allowed placing pressure on or preventing pressure to the abdomen during the various phases of childbirth (ibid. 257ff.). Read did not categorically reject relieving pain through the use of medication, but his experience was that women he tended to did not need it. In his opinion, "the best and safest means of eliminating pain is a properly tuned, controlled inner attitude" (ibid. 133). Read's goal was for child-bearing women to exercise self-discipline, which according to his program they could achieve through information, physical training, and education. In his view, it was the parturient woman who was capable of and should actively influence childbirth.

Read also drew up a four-point catalogue for conducting childbirth for obstetricians (ibid. 157ff.): 1. Patience and being able to wait as well as the midwife's or physician's undivided attention to the woman giving birth. 2. Calmness, so that the women can relax while giving birth and focus on the "occasion [that] demands her full concentration" (Dick-Read 2006: 189). 3. Personal interest, which is meant to give the woman a feeling of security that the physician or midwife is someone on whose knowledge, ability, and judgment she can depend. The woman is also strengthened by someone's mere presence, goodness, and having her hand held. 4. The last point is the physician's close observation of the birth, which is why he or she should stand very close beside the women giving birth. According to read, obstetrics requires more patience and devotion on the part of the physician than hardly any other field. He advocated obstetrical ethics that started out from the assumption that most births had no complications and only in very few cases required intervention. Read understood giving birth as a special life situation that needed personal care in order to exercise a positive influence on the woman to give birth by virtue of her own strength.

His concept exhibited clear parallels to the supervision of home childbirths by midwives, for the midwife was constantly at a woman's side. However, she did not proceed according to a plan but, as Wiebke Lisner writes, ideally supported each woman giving birth, adapting her assistance to the needs of the woman and her family (Lisner 2006: 224).

Read publicly attacked the gynecologist profession with his theses that childbirth was an achievement and that women could experience giving birth without fear and pain, without anesthesia and obstetrical intervention. He considered most of the intervention by his counterparts superfluous, even damaging. Read's criticism of the obstetrics practiced in hospitals made him very unpopular in the special branch of obstetrics, as a report in the magazine *Der Spiegel* of 1955 shows (Der Spiegel, 1.6.1955). In contrast, the monograph he wrote about his childbirth concept and addressed to women flew off the shelves, as will be shown in the following.

CONSCIOUSLY EXPERIENCE CHILDBIRTH AND "SYSTEMATICALLY" CONFRONT LABOR

The book by Dick-Read on "natural childbirth" became a bestseller in numerous industrial countries, including West Germany. The first German translation of the book was published in 1950 with the gripping title *Mutterwerden ohne Schmerz. Die natürliche Geburt.*[9] By 1972, 200,000 copies

---

9   Literally this means "Becoming a mother without pain. Natural childbirth"; the original title of the 1st edition is: Dick-Read, Grantly (1942): Revelation of Childbirth. The principles and practice of natural childbirth, London: Heinemann.

of the guidebook had been published, which was reprinted and amended nineteen times

Read's book explicitly addressed women. He wrote it in a popular style, backing it up with numerous examples from his practice. After 1956, the guidebook was supplemented by a brochure entitled *Der Weg zur natürlichen Geburt. Einführung in die Original Methode Read.*[10] It contained information about the physical processes during pregnancy and childbirth as well as examples of exercises and general advice.

As the magazine *Constanze* reported in 1955, many women acquired the method by reading the book and performed the exercises according to the instructions (Constanze 1955c: 13). Some pregnant women also attended a Read course conducted by a physiotherapist. However, these courses took place only rarely at first, even in large cities (Schumann 2009, 150ff.). The pregnant women paid for the courses themselves until 1972, when a childbirth preparation course became one of the standard medical insurance benefits.

Magazines such as *Constanze* also popularized the Read method. It published two comprehensive articles on the Read birth in 1955 in which mothers also reported on their experience with the method. These reports as well as the letters to the editor written in response constitute the material for the following media analysis.

Constanze popularized the Read method in 1955 as a counter-model to hospital delivery, for at the time, childbirth took place while a woman was unconscious. The concept of "natural" childbirth according to Read and "unconscious" delivery in the hospital, which occurred under the influence of medication and promised women painless childbirth, were contrasted. The debate in the introductory article in *Constanze* contained the following:

Nearly all women are afraid of the pain accompanying childbirth. Of course, a woman can give birth to a baby while under anesthesia. But anesthesia is tricky. Often, childbirth is not easier, but more difficult. And indeed, a woman does not want to be anesthetized during the happiest moment of her life. 'Then I prefer pain,' many

---

10 "The way to natural childbirth. Introduction to the Read-method"; the original title was: Antenatal illustrated. The Natural Approach to Happy Motherhood, 1st ed 1955, London: Heinemann. In 1965, the number of copies reached 53,000, and by 1976 it was more than 100,000.

of those mothers decide who do not want to miss out on this joy. (Constanze 1955a: 98)

Thus, for many women at the time, consciously experiencing childbirth was attractive. "Natural" childbirth was directed toward these women, as, according to the reports in *Constanze,* the method enabled both: a relative lack of pain *and* a conscious experience of childbirth. This wish was fulfilled for Gisela K., for instance, who gave an account of her uncomplicated childbirth after visiting a childbirth preparation course: After learning the method in a gymnastics school, she gave birth to her daughter in the hospital within four hours (Constanze 1955b: 100). In her opinion, this was only possible because she was able to "systematically" face her painful labor, as she summed up the techniques she learned in the course: "Everything— breathing, exercise, relaxation, proper nourishment, comfortable clothing— gives you the feeling of having done everything to simplify the birth for yourself and the baby" (Constanze 1955b: 100). According to this account, Gisela K. had prepared herself for childbirth and had precise ideas about how she would experience it. Based on another report in *Constanze,* however, it becomes evident that the physicians in the delivery room did not necessarily respect women's requests for natural childbirth.

Christel K. therefore did not turn to the nearest hospital, because she knew that they did not like to work according to Read (Constanze 1955c: 13). However, she had heard about "capable senior physician" elsewhere with whom she wanted to deliver her child that way. He was hardly responsive to her questions about the Read method during the brief examinations, yet praised it as "excellent." When Christel K. went into labor and arrived at the hospital, she was greeted by the attending midwife in a very unfriendly way. She told Christel K. that they did not particularly like "gymnasts," because they were always so tense. Yet Christel K. did not allow herself to be discouraged and proceeded according to the Read method. At the last moment, however, the physician came in, and as she moaned, he said: we only want to help you, and placed the anesthesia mask over her mouth and nose. When she woke up out of the brief daze she had already borne her child. Christel K. concludes that,

Not a single one of Dr. Read's valuable insights was put into practice, these physicians and midwives for whom fear and pain continue to be natural side effects of every childbirth, this anesthesia mask that robs the mother of experiencing the birth of her child in an alert state, and this unloving atmosphere in the hospital, which has to make natural, painless childbirth nearly impossible. (Constanze 1955c: 61)

Thus, in the institution of the "hospital," different ideas collided about what methods should be used to relieve the pain of childbirth. At the same time, women giving birth could only apply the Read method in the hospital if physicians and midwives tolerated it. Negotiations took place in the delivery room over who had the prerogative of interpreting what "proper" childbirth is, the women giving birth or the medical experts.

Above and beyond this, the reports show that the various obstetrical concepts about pain relief during childbirth raise further issues. Thus, on a subtle level, the question of women's ability was touched on: were they in a position to deal with childbirth by virtue of their own strength and consciously endure the pain? On the other hand, readers of *Constanze* openly discussed what makes a "good mother." Did women not have the fundamental need to experience the child's first manifestations of life? (Constanze 1955d: 104f.) Does the "first cry" not answer the burning question: is my child alive, and is it healthy? It was here that the reader's opinions differed: women were predominantly prepared to endure pain in order to hear their child's first cry. This apparently tied in with what they expected of a "good mother," who wants to be informed immediately about the state of her child and does not first and foremost think about pain relief. Only one women disagreed: she would hear the child crying often enough and could well go without hearing its first cry. She still considered herself a good mother. Women who made a conscious decision for "unconscious childbirth" were apparently—like the women who consciously decided against one—subject to pressure to justify themselves.

According to the magazine, the numerous letters to the editor about the report in *Constanze* nearly all confirm, that "most gynecologists think little of achieving painless childbirth by means of relaxation exercises and psychological preparation. They prefer the anesthesia mask" (Constanze 1955d: 104). The latter overwhelmingly demonstrated that hospitals did not make sufficient arrangements for women's wish for "natural" childbirth. A lack of time and a lack of interest were the main reasons for not implementing the Read method. The debate furthermore made it apparent that the readers of *Constanze* wanted relatively painless childbirth, and most of them wanted to be completely alert.

MODIFICATION OF THE READ-CONCEPT— ADAPTATION TO CLINICAL OBSTETRICS

In the 1950s, while women were extremely interested in the Read method, the directors of the large women's clinics showed little interested. They preferred the current pharmacological agents. Among physicians, Read's method was thought to be unscientific and the book an "intuitive, empirical" work due to his popular style of writing (Killus 1979: 64). However, obstetricians were forced to look into the Read birth because the press repeatedly took up the issue and women, above all private patients, inquired about the method in hospitals (Interview Hipp 10/19/2001).[11] In order to be able to do justice to these privileged women and offer them, as the midwife Maria Hipp put it, "modern" obstetrical care, the senior physicians of the gynecological hospitals and wards sent their midwives to advanced training courses (Interview Hipp 10/19/2001; Interview Reinke 1/24/2002).[12]

Only individual obstetricians, such as the Hamburg-based gynecologist Rudolf Hellmann, advocated the Read concept in its pure form and used it in their practices (Der Spiegel 1955). Large hospitals, on the other hand, adopted Read's basic ideas about conducting childbirth and adapted his concept to the hospital's framework conditions, such as, for example, the university women's clinic in Tübingen. Beginning in 1957, under the direction of Hans Roemer,[13] the physicians Karl Hermann Lukas and his colleague Probst converted the organization of the supervision of pregnant women and deliveries into so-called "psychological" obstetrics. However, the Tübingen concept, which was published by Lukas in 1959 as a guide for

---

11 Beginning in the mid-1950s, Maria Hipp was the head midwife at the Heidelberg University women's clinic.
12 Annemarie Reinke was head midwife at the women's clinic in Göttingen beginning in 1959.
13 The physician Hans Roemer (1907–1973) began his activity at the Tübingen University women's clinic in 1956, where he introduced the Read childbirth method (Bachmann 1973).

professional people active in the area of obstetrics, deviated from the Readian original on some important points.

The obstetricians did not allow for the continuous individual supervision of a woman giving birth, as in reality there was not always a physician present in the hospital. According to Lukas, there should therefore on no account be a strong bond to the physician (Lukas 1959: 76ff.), which is why he preferred group instruction for preparing women for childbirth.

Thus each course participant is trained to be independent, which is particularly important in a clinic, where the physician who supervised the group cannot be available day and night. Individual preparation always harbors the danger that the pregnant woman lays responsibility for the success of the method on the physician, while group preparation places the focus on a woman's responsibility for herself. (ibid. 77f.)

Lukas saw further advantages in group training in that it allowed saving time and personnel, above all from a psychological point of view (ibid. 72). For the dynamics in the course, which he considered to be a kind of "community of fate," was meant to lead to mutual incentive and self-discipline among the pregnant women. Yet he did not rule out removing a woman from the course if she stood out as being "too loud" or "anxious" and supervise her individually (ibid. 78f.).

In Tübingen, an attempt was made to develop a concept for a method of simplifying childbirth that was compatible with the conditions that prevailed in West German clinics and did not, like the Read method, challenge the strict institutional procedure in the delivery room. Lukas also saw group supervision as an opportunity for women to "educate" each other to "properly" give birth, the physician only occupying a control function. In addition, Lukas also viewed group supervision as a guarantee for propagating the method among the population.

A further difference between Read and the physicians in Tübingen was their attitude toward administering analgesics. While both concepts basically rejected them, according to the Tübingen model, women giving birth were routinely given a local anesthetic when the child's head appeared in order to be able to painlessly treat an episiotomy after childbirth.[14] Lukas considered an episiotomy advisable as a preventive measure, especially for women giving birth for the first time (ibid. 118f.). Because a local anesthetic could only be injected by a physician, this measure required his presence during childbirth. In this way, by applying the "psychological childbirth supervision" developed in Tübingen, obstetrical physicians could present themselves as modern and open-minded, yet indispensable. Because the episiotomy and the routine medication that was injected at the same time reinforced the hierarchical structures in the clinic in favor of the physician. On the other hand, the routine medication also set clear limits to the women's wishes.

An innovation that Read had not allowed for was the conversation with the pregnant woman during a warm-water bath, where women who were not yet familiar with it were given brief instruction in Read's childbirth method. The bath, which was common in the clinic in Tübingen, served to relax the woman and was the force behind it, as the midwife was meant to provide the pregnant woman with information about the birth process during the bath, instruct her in how she should conduct herself, and communicate a feeling of security. According to Lukas, following the brief instruction in the Read method during a warm-water bath, three-fourths of these women succeeded in practicing the method (ibid. 104ff.). The standard for the success of psychological obstetrics was the pregnant woman's self-discipline, which was deduced from the consumption of medication and the duration of childbirth. In his clinical studies, Lukas allowed for four categories of success (ibid. 120ff.). The average result in the Tübingen clinic was "very good" for women "who conducted themselves calmly and disciplined during delivery, for whom, by their own account, the labor pains were tolerable without the aid of medication, and childbirth occurred within a normal amount of time" (ibid. 121).

---

14 The perineal is cut between the vagina and the anus. Obstetrics saw the intervention's benefit in the reduction of overstretching and injury to the mother's soft tissue, the shortening of the expulsive phase, as well as the prevention of descensus of the uterus or the bladder and routinely performed it (Martius 1977: 273). However, the effectivity of the episiotomy has not been scientifically proven (Steffen 2001: 7; Sayn-Wittgenstein 2007: 68f.).

According to Lukas' studies, these were 37 percent of the women. Women in the category "good" differed from those in the first group only in that they required the analgesic meperidine[15]—their share was 43 percent. Fifteen percent of the women in the third group exhibited "moderate success"—they were impatient and restless, quickly insisted on receiving pain relievers, did not implement the breathing exercises they had learned, childbirth lasted longer, and they repeatedly received meperidine. At five percent, those women in the fourth group were

complete failures, women who despite all measures hardly settle down, who throw themselves back and forth on the delivery table, shout uncontrollably, and who cannot be approached either with reassuring consolation or an energetic rebuke. They can for the most part only be calmed down by injecting morphine. Because of their unreasonable conduct, the delivery is protracted and occasionally even has to be completed operatively. (Ibid. 122)

According to Lukas, the results achieved by the obstetricians in Tübingen with the aid of psychological preparation for childbirth were comparable with those at an international level that applied the same categories. The disciplined parturient was "reasonable," while the "unreasonable" parturient was panic-stricken, shouted, and acted indiscriminately (ibid. 61). Gynecologists now judged women giving birth according to their ability to control themselves and classified them accordingly.

The letters to the editor of *Constanze* mentioned above indicate that in the 1950s, women no longer wanted to passively submit themselves to childbirth but were self-determined and wanted to give birth independent of medicine. They wanted the medical aspect to remain in the background. What the letters to the editor also show is by their preparing for childbirth according to the Read method, women expected to get their own room for maneuver in the clinic, which appeared to give them a feeling of sovereignty. The Read concept they learned in the course or read up on provided them with a scheme, a plan toward which they could orient themselves in

---

15 Meperidine was the most widespread analgesic in obstetrics at the time. It was administered rectally or intravenously. It was subject to the German Narcotics Act and could damage the unborn child's respiratory center (Martius/ Gschwendter 1959: 77-80).

the delivery room. Read empowered women giving birth with "instructed self-determination" to organize the birth of their child in a heteronomous framework. Yet his concept was disempowering at the same time, as it laid down standards of conduct for women giving birth that they could either fulfill or at which they could fail. The Read concept set new standards with respect to the discipline and self-responsibility of women giving birth.

The Read method in the delivery room can be interpreted as a technique meant to standardize the conduct of women giving birth and in doing so making the delivery predictable for all of those participating in the birth (Schumann 2009: 147). Midwives who were active at the time report that things proceeded much more calmly with the introduction of preparation for childbirth.[16] According to Read, the shared goal of the midwife and the parturient was to adhere to the rules. It can be assumed that the conversations between the midwife and the woman giving birth now concentrated more on maintaining the techniques, thus largely channeling and standardizing them.

The method could not yet assert itself in the 1950s. It can be assumed that one reason for this is that an active and self-confident woman who wanted to give birth "naturally" called into question the authority of scientific medicine and its representatives. The variations on the original Read concept in West German delivery rooms introduced by physicians can be viewed as testimony to this. Furthermore, the self-determined woman also did not correspond with the concept of a woman at the time, which was defined by the role as housewife and being dependent on a breadwinner (Heinemann 1999; Moeller 1998; Schissler 2001).

In the 1960s, the competition between the Read method and hospital delivery accompanied by the administration of anesthetics ended, as the increased used of local pain relief made anesthesia superfluous and women's strongest argument for "natural" childbirth ceased to apply. As early as in the early 1960s, in psychologically oriented obstetrics, pain relief increasingly receded into the background in favor of "shaping the experience of delivery" (Hellmann 1972: 347ff.)—parallel to the rising social demand for experiences as "inward-oriented consumption" (Schulze 1992: 532ff.). Childbirth was no longer viewed first and foremost as a life-threatening event accompanied by fear, and thus other perspectives found entrance into

---

16 Interview with the midwives Mrs. Brandel and Mrs. Wirth on May 19, 2004.

obstetrics. However, it was not until the mid-1970s that the models based on an orientation toward experience and relationship were gradually propagated in West German clinics.[17] A further aspect of relationship-oriented obstetrics was the presence of husbands or male partners in the delivery room, which was meant to contribute to the humanization of obstetrics. In the 1960s, psychologically oriented obstetrics slowly moved into the delivery room, where it not only supplemented textbook medicine. In 1972, a childbirth preparation course became a health insurance benefit if a physician prescribed it as a measure for a pregnant woman.

FROM MIDWIFERY TO OBSTETRICS

In the 1960s, obstetrics was marked by a technological thrust that fundamentally altered the perspective with respect to childbirth and its supervision (Hillemanns 1995; Schmidt-Matthiesen 1988). Prior to that, it was only possible to monitor the fetus by listening to its heart tones with a heart tone stethoscope. A further indication of its state was provided by the color of the amniotic fluid. In the early 1960s, advances in medical and laboratory technology now enabled examining the unborn child in the womb (Schmidt-Matthiesen 1988: 2ff.). Several techniques were available to medicine—fetal blood analysis, cardiotocography (CTG), ultrasound scanners—that allowed direct access to the fetus. The physician's focus on the pregnant woman and her well-being therefore faded, and his obstetrical activity was from now on directed toward the fetus's objective measurement data (Duden 1991; Schindele 1996). This transition as a result of the technologization changed the conception physicians had of themselves in the delivery room. Traditional obstetricians with an observant attitude forfeited their interpretation of the birth to modern, technologically oriented obstetrical physicians (Schumann 2009: 176ff.). The new experts in the area of medical technology, the perinatologists, defined childbirth within the

---

17 What became very popular was the gentle childbirth approach developed by Frederic Leboyer, who gave priority to the child about to be born and the mother-child relationship. Part of his concept, for example, was the rooming in of mother and child, breastfeeding the child immediately after its birth, and breastfeeding on demand (Killus 1979: 12, 29-32).

framework of an epidemiological risk model (Arney 1982; Duden 1998). They judged the safety of childbirth according to statistically defined average values, which formed the basis for the preventive risk control of the birth. Future risks related to the state of the fetus were calculated with the aid of technical equipment and diagnostic calculations performed in the laboratory (Weir 2006). With the technologization of the delivery room, this became the actual object of obstetrics. Until 1975, monitoring procedures progressively became an element of standard care, which by way of the maternity guidelines became a standard health insurance benefit for women, most recently the ultrasound examination in 1972 (Schmidt-Matthiesen 1988: 4). The consolidation of monitoring and control by experts resulted in increasing intervention in childbirth: according to obstetrical physician Schmidt-Matthiesen, "the trend toward the precautionary prevention of harm" meant that in the mid-1950s, the number of Cesarean sections rose from three to four percent, and in the mid-1980s from 15 to 20 percent. According to Schmidt-Matthiesen, for obstetrical physicians, the progress of the development outlined lay in the fact that obstetrics had lost its emergency character, as the large volume of information gained through the use of technology made obstetrics a "discipline that takes preventive action."

The technological possibilities of monitoring childbirth profoundly changed obstetrics, and this led to a "restructuring of obstetrics" (Käser 1967) in the mid-1960s. In the process, the representatives of classic obstetrics were ousted by the proponents of technical obstetrics. The newly forming subdiscipline of perinatology, with its protagonist Erich Saling, made sole claim to performing modern and safe obstetrics by means of technological diagnostics.[18] This process of professionalization was accompanied by media campaigns in which the representatives of technological obstetrics attacked traditional obstetricians: because of their backwardness, they bore sole responsibility for the high maternal and infant mortality rates (Neuhauser 1969: 26,130f.). The demands made by obstetrical physicians concentrated on furnishing delivery rooms with technical equipment, staff

---

18 Erich Saling (1925), a Berlin-based gynecologist, directed the obstetrical ward at the municipal women's clinic in Berlin-Neukölln from 1976 to 1991. He is regarded as an eminent authority in his field even beyond Germany's borders (http://www.saling-institut.de/german/02saling/02cv.html [accessed on June 16, 2006]), see Lenzen 1991: 45.

sufficiently trained in modern childbirth technology, and the regionalization or centralization of obstetrical clinics and their provisions for emergencies (Saling 1967). With the introduction of obstetrics oriented toward preventive medical technology, obstetrical medicine at the same time legitimized its sole authority to oversee childbirth and in the mid-1960s declared childbirth to be the "most high-risk period of a woman's life" (Eirich 2003). West German healthcare policymakers supported the expansion of perinatology based on the argument that technological methods reduced maternal and infant mortality (Lenzen 1991: 39f.). Obstetric-technological perinatological practices also did not give rise to public protest, probably facilitated by the thrust in technological progress that prevailed in society at the time (Döring-Manteuffel 2000; Schildt 2000).

PROGRAMMED CHILDBIRTH

In the course of this transition, obstetrical physicians developed a new method for making childbirth safer, in which the synthetically producible hormone oxytocin, which increases contraction of the uterus during labor, played a primary role. This hormone allowed accelerating childbirth if there were complications, or inducing labor if pregnancy lasted beyond the scheduled due date. It was in emergency situation such as these that physicians used the labor-inducing agent. In the late 1950s, oxytocin enabled "forcing childbirth without harming the child or endangering the mother" (Müller 1960: 68). Labor could now be induced artificially and the intensity and frequency of contractions controlled (Müller 1960). In the mid-1960s, this possibility gave rise to obstetrical physicians inducing labor even without a medical indication (Vogt-Hägerbäumer 1985: 80) from a preventive point of view. This practice, which was developed in the United States (Simmer 1978), became known as "programmed childbirth" in West Germany, but was also referred to as "timed" or "scheduled" childbirth by obstetricians.

It was in particular large women's clinics in big cities that tested the concept of programmed childbirth between the mid-1960s and mid-1970s. The procedure was standardized and was similar to the model used at the Freiburg University women's clinic (Hillemanns 1978c: 26ff.). According to this plan, pregnant women were summoned to the clinic at 5:00 p.m. on the day before the scheduled delivery (1978c: 37f.). An anamnesis was prepared, a CTG performed, the pelvic score ascertained, and in some cases an amnioscopy was performed to control the color of the amniotic fluid. At 9:00 p.m. the pregnant woman was given a sedative injection so that she was rested for the delivery on the following day. She was awakened at 4:45 a.m. the next morning, and at 5:15 a.m. taken into the delivery room, where she was shaved, received an enema, and took a shower. At 5:45 she laid down on the delivery table, was injected with an analgesic, and hooked up to the CTG. At 6:00 a.m. the physician administered the labor-inducing agent and performed an amniotomy at 6:15. This was followed by the administration of a pain reliever as well as a local anesthetic. Depending on the indication, that is, according to the CTG curve, further examinations were performed on the fetus. If childbirth had not yet taken place after six to eight expulsive pains, the child was retrieved per vacuum extraction.[19]

At the Martin Luther Hospital in Berlin, between 1971 and 1976 nearly every fifth women gave birth to her child according to the programmed childbirth model (Stark 1976: 61). At Bremen's general hospital, in 1975 every second birth was induced (Der Spiegel, 1984).

The concept aimed at planning childbirth at its "ideal" moment (Hillemann 1978; Frasch 1987: 81ff.). Whereas childbirth was considered to be on schedule between the 282nd and the 295th day of pregnancy,[20] a pregnancy that lasted longer than 295 days was "postterm," because the placenta begins to deteriorate and the unborn child is no longer supplied with sufficient oxygen (Martius1962: 296f.). If a pregnancy was determined to be postterm, it was considered a risk and in most cases terminated, either by inducing labor artificially or performing a Cesarean section.

Obstetricians oriented toward preventive medicine not only considered the planned inducement of labor to be an advantage in cases of risk pregnancy, this method now also aimed at "optimizing delivery of the so-called normal pregnancy" (Jung 1978: 4f.). Programming childbirth was based on the consideration that the point in time of the beginning of spontaneous birth neither meant that the fetus had achieved ideal maturity nor that it cor-

---

19 In this delivery operation, a ventouse is placed on the child's head and the child is extracted with the aid of a vacuum.
20 Determination of the delivery date was carried out according to the "extended Naegele rule" (Martius 1977: 100).

responded with the ideal state of the placenta's capacity. Obstetrics believed that the physiological beginning of childbirth was only "coincidental"—that is, it did not follow any laws—and was therefore "fundamentally deficient" (Hillemanns 1978a: 1). It believed that nature could be optimized with the aid of science and technology. Using the argument that this lowered the perinatal mortality and morbidity rates, perinatologists began conceiving of childbirth as a program and putting this concept into practice (Martius 1977: 228).

Among physicians, the organizational aspects of scheduled childbirth were a further advantage: the concept was intended to ideally prepare the pregnant woman, her family, and the hospital staff for the upcoming birth (Hillemanns 1978a). In contrast, they saw "childbirth that occurred unexpectedly" as a burden for everyone involved. A scheduled delivery date enabled pregnant women to coordinate their family, arrange for their other children to be taken care of, and to arrange the household accordingly (Richter 1978). Physicians also thought it was useful in that the husband could fit the date of birth into his working rhythm and accompany his wife from the start. In addition, doctors also propagated a psychological benefit for the woman: these preparations would make it possible for her to face childbirth calmly.

In practice, in the 1960s, only those women came into question for programmed childbirth in clinics in large cities who had personally called on the hospital during pregnancy, been examined there, and arranged a delivery date. Women who went to the clinic and were already experiencing labor pains were excluded. Pregnant women summoned to the clinic for programmed childbirth were often private patients and had a right to be treated and her baby delivered by a senior physician. However, senior physicians attached great weight to their personal ties with their privileged private patients. These pregnant women were also disappointed if the senior physician who accompanied their pregnancies did not perform the delivery himself, as the Freiburg obstetrician Hans-Günter Hillemanns stated. In the Freiburg University women's clinic he directed, two-thirds of the programmed deliveries he supervised were performed on private patients (Hillemanns 1978d), because this form of delivery required a great deal of obstetrical experience (Interview Hipp 10/19/2001).

Gynecologists evaluated the arguments in favor of programmed childbirth differently. Whereas some placed emphasis on the safety aspect for the child, others considered the organizational reasons to be more decisive. Another legitimate reason was that assisting childbirth was to take place during working hours (Hillemanns 1978c).

However, in the mid-1970s, when the social acceptance of programming childbirth declined (Stark 1976), obstetricians did not expect an improvement in the obstetrical results in terms of a concept, but conceded that "we can definitely be satisfied if we achieve the same good results as during a well-supervised spontaneous birth" (Baumgarten as quoted in Hillemanns 1978c: 25). Based on their prior experience, they saw the decisive advantages in the area of organization (Schmidt/Dudenhausen/Saling 1978). In doing so, the obstetrical experts underscored the fact that the organization of bearing children with the aid of medicinal and technological developments had first and foremost meant planning security for all of those involved.

With programmed childbirth, the perinatologists had tied in with the general concepts of planning and feasibility that had prevailed in the 1960s. As a planned occurrence, the commencement of birth, into which was intervened only if there were complications, not only promised more safety, but could be better integrated into a woman's and her family's everyday life. Obstetricians banked on lessening the fear of the woman giving birth through knowledge of the date and the timing of childbirth. At the same time, the program meant that optimum care could be provided in hospital. From the viewpoint of obstetrics, planning security had a positive effect in this respect. For those doctors participating in the birth, it solved the problem of constantly being on standby—prior to that, gynecologists had to interrupt their daily routines when they were summoned to "unplanned" spontaneous births (Hillemanns 1978b).

Programmed childbirth constituted the culmination of the rationalization phase in obstetrics. Bearing a child was conceived as a planned and preventive process in which all of the risks seemed to be calculable and could therefore—according to the obstetrical understanding at the time—be minimized.

In the mid-1970s, the concept of programmed childbirth began to be criticized by the women's movement. Under the motto "My belly belongs to me" it demanded sexual self-determination and assumed a "radical stance" on gynecology and clinical obstetrics within the scope of a general critique of technology and medicine (Sperling 1994; Stolzenberg 2000). For the women's movement, safety was not guaranteed by obstetrics geared toward planning, but one that was geared toward human needs (Stark 1976).

This signaled the end of an epoch for obstetrics that was marked by unrestrained progress and planning euphoria as well as trust in technological solutions, and there began, haltingly at first, a phase of the pluralization of obstetrical choices. Due to the public pressure of the women's movement, obstetrics gradually shifted its guiding principles from programmed childbirth to "human, family-oriented obstetrics," without, however, reducing individual practices—such as, for example, controlling childbirth by artificially inducing labor. On the contrary: they steadily advanced the medicalization of giving birth (Schwartz/Schücking 2002).

Conclusions

In the 1950s and 1960s, obstetrics in the Federal Republic of Germany was transformed and scientized through the hospitalization of births. Childbirth in the hospital became something accessible from the outside. In the process, the foundation for the care of women giving birth changed. While the conventional practice had previously aimed for the continuous social supervision of the midwife, in the institution of the clinic this orientation gave way to the supervision of childbirth according to a standardized program.

In the opinion of obstetrical experts, two obstetrical methods with different scientific justifications—the Read model of childbirth and the model of programmed childbirth—were to make giving birth more efficient and more tolerable as well as heighten the safety of delivery in the clinic. Whereas the two concepts initially seemed to be opposing trends, they both corresponded to the zeitgeist of planning and developed side by side. The protagonists of these childbirth models, Read and Saling, were both initially outsiders in their fields. Each of them attempted to optimize obstetrics by means of a control model—the one through a model based on planning in advance, the other through one that had a mental influence. The Read method addressed the pregnant woman with information and education—by means of the schematic application of acquired knowledge, she was to actively promote the birth of her child in the sense of "guided" self-determination. In contrast, the concept of programmed birth aimed at the physician's activity. While technological obstetrics preventively controlled childbirth from the outside, according to the Read concept the woman giving birth was in command. Both concepts initially reached privileged private patients, who shared the notions of the necessity of a careful and planned approach to childbirth with the physicians. Neither Read nor Saling viewed giving birth as a natural process, but as one that could be influenced socially. With his concept of "natural" childbirth, Grantly Dick-Read may have made rhetorical reference to "nature"—however, his concept of childbirth was defined by the predominant zeitgeist of planning, as was programmed childbirth. Yet while both concepts were consistent with social norms, they interpreted them differently: programmed childbirth went hand in hand with a belief in progress and technology, and the Read method addressed women's self-determination and ability. On the one hand, their methods and directions are at opposite poles, yet on the other hand, they feature an internal connection through their anticipatory, planning organization of the course of childbirth. The two childbirth models, both of which aim toward planning, changed the relationship between midwife and the woman giving birth in hospital, where the midwife had to monitor the adherence to standards, making it hardly possible to pay attention to the woman giving birth.

However, whether a childbirth model attains social acceptance is decisively determined by the actors in the area of health policy.

Translation by Rebecca van Dyke

REFERENCES

Arney, William Ray (1982): Power and the profession of obstetrics, Chicago: University of Chicago Press.
Bachmann, F. (1973): "Nachruf für Hans Roemer", in: Deutsche Hebammenzeitschrift 25, p. 225.
Beske, Fritz (1958): "Zur Soziologie der Haus- und Klinikentbindungen", in: Deutsche Hebammenzeitschrift 10, pp. 157-160.
Beske, Fritz (1967): "Die Hebamme in Gegenwart und Zukunft", in: Deutsche Hebammenzeitschrift 19, pp. 453-456.

Constanze (1955a): "Turnstunde mit Constanze. Geburt ohne Angst", in: Constanze, 8/12/1955, pp. 98-99.
— (1955b): "Ich habe natürlich entbunden" in: Constanze, 8/12/1955, p. 100.
— (1955c): "Geburten im alten Trott", in: Constanze, 8/20/1955, pp.13, 60-61.
— (1955d): "Mütter und Hebammen schrieben zum Thema: Geburten im alten Trott", in: Constanze, 8/24/1955, pp. 104-105.
Declercq, Eugene et al (2001): "Where to give birth? Politics and the place of birth", in: Raymond DeVries/Cecilia Benoit/Edwin R. van Teijlingen/Sirpa Wrede (eds), Birth by design. Pregnancy, maternity care, and midwifery in North America and Europe, New York: Routledge, pp. 7-27.
Dick-Read, Grantly (1960): Mutterwerden ohne Schmerz. Die natürliche Geburt, Hamburg: Hoffmann & Campe
— (1972): Mutterwerden ohne Schmerz. Die natürliche Geburt, Hamburg: Hoffmann & Campe.
— (1978): Der Weg zur natürlichen Geburt. Mit Übungsbeispielen, Hamburg: Hoffmann & Campe.
— (2006): Childbirth without fear, London: Pollinger Limited.
Döring-Manteuffel, Anselm (ed) (2006): Strukturmerkmale der deutschen Geschichte des 20. Jahrhunderts, assisted by Elisabeth Müller-Luckner, Munich: Oldenbourg.
Duden, Barbara (1991): Der Frauenleib als öffentlicher Ort. Vom Missbrauch des Begriffs Leben, Munich: Deutscher Taschenbuch.
— (1998): "Die Ungeborenen. Vom Untergang der Geburt im späten 20. Jahrhundert", in: Jürgen Schlumbohm/Barbara Duden/Jaques Gélis/Patrice Veit (eds), Rituale der Geburt. Eine Kulturgeschichte. Munich: C.H.Beck, pp. 149-169.
Eirich, Martina (2003): "Wichtig war, dass jeder wagte zu sagen, was er dachte", Martina Eirich im Gespräch mit Prof. Alfred Rockenschaub; available at http://www.geburtskanal.de/Wissen/G/GeburtshilfeRockenschaub.v. php (last accessed 1/7/2011).
Fitzek, Josef (1957): Über die Einstellung der Frau zur klinischen und häuslichen Geburtshilfe; unpublished doctoral thesis, University of Cologne.
Frasch, Gisela (1987): Die Frage Hausgeburt/Klinikentbindung vor ihrem historischen und aktuellen Hintergrund. Dissertation im Fach Medizin

an der Frauenklinik und -poliklinik im Klinikum Charlottenburg der Freien Universität Berlin, Berlin: Hochschulschrift Freie Universität Berlin.

Goecke, Hermann (1962): Gestaltwandel in der Gynäkologie und Geburtshilfe in den letzten 35 Jahren, Münster: Aschendorff.

Grabrucker, Marianne (1996): Vom Abenteuer der Geburt. Die letzten Landhebammen erzählen, Frankfurt a.M.: Fischer-Taschenbuch.

Grubenmann, Ottilia (1993/1995): 200 Praxisfälle, vols. 1 and 2, 2nd edition. Weissbad: Alpstein.

HebG (1938):Hebammengesetz vom 21.12.1938, in: RGBl., I, p. 1893.

HebG (1954): Hebammengesetz vom 4. Januar 1954, in: BGBl. p. 1.

Heineman, Elisabeth (1999): What difference does a husband make? Women and material status in Nazi and postwar Germany, Berkeley: University of California Press.

Hellmann, Rudolf (1972): "Nachwort", in: Dick-Read 1972.

Henze, Ricarda (1999): Geburtshilfe in den 50er und 60er Jahren in Niedersachsen aus Sicht der damals freien Hebammen; unpublished diploma thesis, University of Hanover.

Hillemanns, Hans-Günter (ed) (1978): Die programmierte Geburt. 1. Freiburger geburtshilfliches Kolloquium 1976, Stuttgart, Thieme.

— (1978a): "Einleitung", in: Hans-Günter Hillemanns (1978), pp. 1-3.

— (1978b): "Auswahlkriterien: Organisation der Geburtshilfe als Indikation", in: Hans-Günter Hillemanns (1978), pp. 19-22.

— (1978c): "Zu den Methoden der Geburtseinleitung bei programmierter Geburt", in: Hans-Günter Hillemanns (1978), pp. 26-51.

— (1978d): "Abschließende Diskussion", in: Hans-Günter Hillemanns (1978), pp. 132-140.

— (ed) (1995): Geburtshilfe—Geburtsmedizin. Eine umfassende Bilanz zukunftsweisender Entwicklungen am Ende des 20. Jahrhunderts, Berlin: Springer.

Jung, H. (1978): "Definition, Motivation, Entwicklung", in: Hans-Günter Hillemanns (1978), pp. 3-8.

Käser, O. (1967): "Einleitendes Referat zum Podiumsgespräch über die Neuordnung der Geburtshilfe", 36. Versammlung der Deutschen Gesellschaft für Gynäkologie vom 20.-24. 9.1966, in: Archiv für Gynäkologie 204(2 and 3), pp. 298-301.

Killus, Jürgen (1979): Geburtsmethoden. Eine vergleichende Studie. Vol. 1. Leboyer, Lamaze, Dick-Read, Programmierte Geburt, Stuttgart: Windhüter.

Lenzen, Dieter (1991): Krankheit als Erfindung. Medizinische Eingriffe in die Kultur, Frankfurt a.M.: Fischer-Taschenbuch.

Lindner, Ulrike (2004): Gesundheitspolitik in der Nachkriegzeit. Großbritannien und die Bundesrepublik Deutschland im Vergleich, München: Oldenbourg.

Linner, Rosalie (1989): Tagebuch einer Landhebamme 1943-1980, 2nd ed, Rosenheim: Rosenheimer.

Lisner, Wiebke (2006): "Hüterinnen der Nation." Hebammen im Nationalsozialismus, Frankfurt a.M.: Campus.

Loytved, Christine (2004): "Geduld in der Geburtshilfe aus historischer Perspektive", in: Die Hebamme 17, pp. 18-21.

Lukas, Karl Hermann (1959): Die psychologische Geburtserleichterung. Anleitung für Ärzte, Hebammen und Krankengymnastinnen zur psychologischen Geburtsvorbereitung und Geburtsleitung, 1st ed, Stuttgart: Schattauer.

Martius, Gerhard/Gschwendter, Rita (1959): Die Vorbereitung auf die Geburt. Eine Anleitung für werdende Mütter, Munich: Reinhardt.

Martius, Gerhard (1962): "Der regelwidrige Verlauf von Schwangerschaft, Geburt und Wochenbett", in: Werner Bickenbach (ed), Hebammenlehrbuch, Stuttgart: Thieme pp. 265-395.

— (1977): "Regelwidrige Schwangerschaftsdauer", in: Gerhard Martius (ed), Lehrbuch der Geburtshilfe. Für die Ausbildung des Studenten. Für die Weiterbildung des Arztes. Mit Lernzielangaben und 115 Prüfungsfragen, Stuttgart: Thieme, pp. 213-232.

Moeller, Robert, G. (1997): Geschützte Mütter. Frauen und Familien in der westdeutschen Nachkriegspolitik. Trans. Heidrun Homburg, Munich: Deutscher Taschenbuch.

Müller, H.A. (1960): "Symposium über Oxytozin in Montevideo vom 17.-19.8.1959", in: Geburtshilfe und Frauenheilkunde 20, pp. 65-71.

Neuhauser, Peter (1969): "Das Risiko, in Deutschland geboren zu werden", in: Der Stern, 22/27/1969, pp. 16-26, 131-132.

Niehuss, Merith (2001): Familie, Frau und Gesellschaft: Studien zur Strukturgeschichte der Familien in Westdeutschland 1945-1960, Göttingen: Vandenhoeck & Ruprecht.

Olbrich, Katrin (1996): Die Schmerzarme Geburt im ersten Drittel des 20. Jahrhunderts im deutschen Sprachraum. Ihre Beziehung zum Frauenbild der Gynäkologen und zum Geburtenrückgang; unpublished doctoral thesis, University of Greifswald.

Richter, D. (1978): "Psychohygienische Aspekte bei programmierter Geburt", in: Hans-Günter Hillemanns (1978), pp. 22-24.

Saling, Erich (1967): "Vorschläge zur Neuordnung der Geburtshilfe", in: Geburtshilfe und Frauenheilkunde 27(6), pp. 572-585.

Sayn-Wittgenstein zu, Friederike (ed) (2007): Geburtshilfe neu denken. Bericht zur Situation und Zukunft des Hebammenwesens in Deutschland, Bern: Huber.

Scherer, Richard (1970): Klinikgeburt, Hausgeburt, Situation der Hebamme in Mittel- und Oberfranken; unpublished doctoral thesis, University of Erlangen-Nuremberg.

Schindele, Eva (1996): Pfusch an der Frau. Krankmachende Normen. Überflüssige Operationen. Lukrative Geschäfte, Frankfurt a.M.: Fischer.

Schildt, Axel (2000): "Materieller Wohlstand-pragmatische Politik-kulturelle Umbrüche. Die 60er Jahre in der Bundesrepublik", in: Axel Schildt/Detlef Siegfried/Christian Lammers (eds), Dynamische Zeiten: die 60er Jahre in den beiden deutschen Gesellschaften, Hamburg: Christians, pp. 21-53.

Schissler, Hanna (2001): "'Normalisation' as project. Some thoughts on gender relations in West Germany during the 1950s", in: Hanna Schissler (ed), The Miracle Years. A Cultural History of West Germany, 1949-1968, Princeton: Princeton University Press, pp. 359-375.

Schmidt, Eberhardt/Dudenhausen, Joachim W./Saling, Erich (1978): "Podiumsgespräch: Vor- und Nachteile der sogenannten programmierten Geburt", in: Perinatale Medizin, vol. VII. 8. Deutscher Kongress für Perinatale Medizin Berlin 3.-7. Mai 1977, Stuttgart: Thieme, pp. 416-418.

Schmidt-Matthiesen, H. (1988): Wandlungen. Die Entwicklung der Gynäkologie von 1948–1988. Eine kritische Bilanz. Farewell lecture held by Prof. Dr. H. Schmidt-Matthiesen on February 8, 1988, at the Frankfurt am Main University Women's Clinic, Munich: Urban und Schwarzenberg.

Schulze, Gerhard (1992): Die Erlebnisgesellschaft: Kultursoziologie der Gegenwart, Frankfurt a.M.: Campus.

Schumann, Marion (2006): "Westdeutsche Hebammen zwischen Hausgeburtshilfe und klinischer Geburtsmedizin", in: Bund Deutscher Hebammen e.V. (ed), Zwischen Bevormundung und beruflicher Autonomie. Die Geschichte des Bundes Deutscher Hebammen, Karlsruhe: Hippokrates, pp. 113-173.

— (2009): Vom Dienst an Mutter und Kind zum Dienst nach Plan. Hebammen in der Bundesrepublik 1950–1975, Göttingen: V&R Uni-Press.

Schwarz, Clarissa M./Schücking, Beate A. (2004): "Adieu, normale Geburt? Ergebnisse eines Forschungsprojekts", in: Dr. med. Mabuse, 29 (148), pp. 22-25.

Simmer, H.-H. (1978): "Zur Geschichte der Programmierten Geburt", in: Eberhard Schmidt/Joachim Wolfram Dudenhausen/Erich Saling (eds), Perinatale Medizin. 8. Deutscher Kongress für Perinatale Medizin, Berlin, 3.–7. Mai 1977, pp. 413-415.

Simon, Michael (2000): Krankenhauspolitik in der Bundesrepublik Deutschland. Historische Entwicklung und Probleme der politischen Steuerung stationärer Versorgung, Opladen: Westdeutscher.

Sperling, Urte (1994): "Schwangerschaft und Medizin. Zur Genese und Geschichte der Medikalisierung des weiblichen Gebärvermögens", in: Reinhard Busse et al (ed): Gesundheitskult und Krankheitswirklichkeit, Hamburg: Argument, pp. 7-21.

Der Spiegel (1955): "Read. Geburt ist Arbeit", in: Der Spiegel, 9/23/1955, pp. 30-37.

Der Spiegel (1984): "Geburtshilfe: Fahrerflucht im Kreißsaal"; available at http://www.spiegel.de/spiegel/print/d-13513537.html (last accessed 1/7/2011).

Springborn, Anne (1964): "Es brennt in allen Ecken", in: Deutsche Hebammenzeitschrift, 16, p. 204.

Stark, Eva-Maria (1976): Geboren werden und Gebären. Eine Streitschrift für die Neugestaltung von Schwangerschaft, Geburt und Mutterschaft, Munich: Frauenoffensive.

Steffen, Gisèle (2001): Ist der routinemäßige, prophylaktische Dammschnitt gerechtfertigt? Überblick über neuere Forschungsarbeiten, Trans. Monika Gepperth, 5th ed, Frankfurt a.M.: Mabuse.

Stolzenberg, Regina (1998): "Die Sehnsucht nach Ganzheit und Gleichheit. Einige Fragen und Antworten zur Standortbestimmung der Frauengesundheitsbewegung", in: Sozialwissenschaftliche Forschung und Praxis für Frauen e.V. (ed), Beiträge zur feministischen Theorie und Praxis. Gesundheitsnormen und Heilsversprechen, 21/49/50 pp. 15-34.

Vogt-Hägerbäumer, Barbara (1985): Schwangerschaft ist eine Erfahrung, die die Frau, den Mann und die Gesellschaft angeht. Probleme beim Kinderkriegen – Lösungen für Frauen und ihre Partner. Reinbek bei Hamburg: Rowohlt.

Weir, Lorna (2006): "Folgen des Risikofaktors", in: Deutsche Hebammenzeitschrift 58, pp. 53-56.

Zimdars, Kurt/Sauer Karl (1955): Erläuterungen zum Hebammengesetz vom 21. Dezember 1938 nebst Gesetz zur Regelung von Fragen des Hebammenwesens vom 4. Januar 1954. Revised and supplemented 3rd edition by Dr. Friedrich Koch and Dr. Fritz Bernhardt, Ministerialräte im Bundesministerium des Innern 1955, Hanover: Staude.

Planning death: Debates on euthanasia, end of life care and living wills in Germany since the 1970s

ISABELLA JORDAN

> Neither my birth nor my death can appear to me as experiences of my own . . . . I can . . . apprehend myself only as 'already born' and 'still alive'—I can apprehend my birth and my death only as prepersonal horizons.
> MAURICE MERLEAU-PONTY

Public debates on dying have been conducted in Germany since the late 1960s, making an issue of the medical and institutional circumstances under which people in Germany die. A prevalent topic within these debates has been the bio-ethical model of "self-determined dying," understood largely as being able to arrange or even plan the phase of dying, either through voluntary euthanasia or through hospice work and palliative medicine. Until recently, debates about death and dying in Germany were conducted by two diametrically opposed movements, one calling for the legalization of euthanasia, the other for hospices and palliativ care. While both movements referred to the concept of self-determination, they filled this concept with different meanings: for the one it meant that individuals are entitled to legally take advantage of euthanasia if they so wish, for the other it meant that people have access to hospices and palliative care when they need it. In this chapter, I will argue, that in the past few years however, these two formerly disparat movements have converged on the point of living wills. This shift of focus towards the issue of the living will has been accompanied by an increasing demand on people, by both movements, to deal with their own dying, to visualize it, to speak about it, and then plan and arrange it.

In the past few years, public debate has been closely interlaced with the issue of the living will, at the latest since 2003. The living will, today, is widely seen as the most important instrument to exercise self-determination in dying. This shift was prompted by a landmark decision by the *Bundesgerichtshof* (Federal Court of Justice) in March 2003. The court for the first time ruled that under certain circumstances it may be admissible to take into account the presumed will of a person who formerly had expressed that he or she did not wish to be kept alive under certain circumstances (Bundesgerichtshof 2003). Previously, there had been a consensus among physicians and legal experts that physicians' duty is "prolonging life at all costs". Since then, public debates on dying have strongly focused on the issue of the living will. So-called living wills can be drawn up as a written expression of someone's wish in case he or she is no longer capable of articulating his or her own will in a possible later state of unconsciousness (Bundesjustizministerium 2010: 2).

The discussion surrounding living wills and their statutory basis has persisted in Germany since the 1960s (May et al 2005: 9). According to May et al, the demand for living wills arose because patients and their families were unsure how a good decision could be made for another person who was incapable of making a decision for him- or herself. Also, May tells us, the demand arose "due to a lack of knowledge about or insecurity with respect to the legal situation, in case of doubt many physicians do everything that is medically possible, or may even orient their range of treatment toward the financial budget of their practice or their hospital ward" (May et al 2005: 9). This view, May argues, is shared by the German Ethics Council's 2005 recommendations on *Patientenverfügung, ein Instrument der Selbstbestimmung* (Living Will, an Instrument of Self-Determination):

The National Ethics Council believes that a person capable of making decisions must, should he or she later be incapable of making a decision for him- or herself, have the right to specify his or her wish for or against later medical treatment. This shall also include the performance or interruption of medically indicated life-sustaining measures or refraining therefrom; in no way, however, shall it include active euthanasia. (May et al 2005: 221)[1]

In contemporary public discourse, the living will is mostly discussed as a means to curb medical paternalism in favor of patient autonomy, the latter being largely understood as "making a decision for him- or herself".

The longstanding controversial discussion about the meaning, the range, as well as the binding character of living wills led in September 2009 to the revision of the *Betreuungsgesetz* (Guardianship Law). Today, under specific circumstances, in health-related matters a patient's written will shall take precedence over the assessment of the attending physician, members of the family, the guardian, or authorized representative (Drittes Gesetz zur Änderung des Betreuungsrechts [Third Statute for the Revision of the Guardianship Law]; on the controversial discussion, see Sahm 2006; Zypries 2007; Bauer 2006). Thus, since September 2009, the living will is of increased significance: the provision laid down in the Third Statute for the Revision of the Guardianship Law allows for restriction or interruption of therapy if the patient is no longer capable of making a clearly articulated decision but has left a written will that he or she wishes termination of medical care in case of a precisely defined situation.

In this contribution I will show that the concepts, goals and values of the euthanasia and the hospice movement which have formerly been mutually exclusive and diametrically opposed to each other, in recent years have apparently converged to a certain extent. Against the background of a previous study of mine, I find this change irritating. In this study, I examined the objectives, motives, courses, blockades, and promotion of the active euthanasia and the hospice movement in Germany and the Netherlands between 1970 and circa 2000. The study looks at the structural and material resources of the movements and analyzes certain key frames with the aid of frame analysis (Jordan 2007). One of the results was that although for both movements, self-determination in dying formed a strong point of reference, it meant very different things. Until approximately 2000, the positions within the debate were divided among advocates of the legal regulation of active euthanasia on the one hand, and opponents thereof on the other.

---

1   All quotations in this chapter have been translated from the German original by Rebecca van Dyck.

There was a clear reference to patient autonomy or self-determination in both positions, yet upon closer examination the standpoints diverged. Certainly, "self-determination in dying" formed a familiar, wide-spread and positively connotated expression to which both movements could refer to. However, at the same time they were filled with very different meaning. For the one camp, it meant that only people whose needs are met and who are cared for attentively are in self-determined circumstances, for the other it meant that people are allowed to select the manner and moment of death with the active involvement of third persons.[2]

SOCIAL BACKGROUND OF THE DEBATES ON DYING

What are the historical developments behind the death debates? Until the mid-20th century, most people in Germany died at home in their familiar environment (Nationaler Ethikrat 2006: 38-41). There are no statistics on where people die in Germany; however, hospital statistics show that in 1953, 37.4 percent of the population died in hospitals. While this number increased in the following years, culminating in 1977 with 55.4 percent, it has been declining since. There are no figures on the number of people who die in nursing homes, so that one can only approximate statistics about the places of death in Germany. According to estimates by the *Statistisches Bundesamt* (Federal Statistical Office), 60 percent of the population die in hospitals and nursing institutions, and circa 40 percent at home (Statistisches Bundesamt 2010). Other sources speak of an 80 percent share of the population who would prefer dying at home rather than in a nursing institution (Student 2009: 4; Gronemeyer 2007: 67).

In the 1960s, new technologies were introduced in intensive medicine that sustained the lives of people who would otherwise have died as a result of their illness. However, this meant that the dying increasingly entered the scope of responsibility of the hospital, resulting in a hospitalization of dy-

---

2 In this study, among other things, I examine the development and the inner dynamics of the German hospice movement and the key frames used by the actors. I show that the demand for self-determination in the final phase of one's life is a motif that is widely discussed and cited by different actors, however it is interpreted in very different ways (Jordan 2007).

ing (Illich 1995: 139; Ariès 1995: 786f; Gronemeyer 2007: 69). Intensive medicine, in particular the heart-lung apparatus, engendered new means of extending life, and first attempts were made to create artificial organs, such as the "artificial heart." In 1968, the Ad hoc Committee of the Harvard Medical School to Examine the Definition of Brain Death recommended brain-death as a new death criterion. The brain-death concept ultimately replaced the cardiovascular death criterion that had prevailed up to that point (Schlich et al 2001: 11), also because it created space for transplantation medicine, that is, removing organs from brain-dead patients and implanting them in patients in need of a new one.[3] It appeared to be possible to prolong life and renew or even replace organs.

In view of developments in medical technology, this progress euphoria is being taken to the extremes by a group of scientists who aim for a range of primarily medical-technical interventions in order to advance the abolishment of aging all the way to overcoming death. Their ideas range from so-called anti-aging medicine, enhancement, and transhumanistic utopias, "delaying death" with the aid of the cryopreservation of the dead or their brains, to abolishing death altogether (see Bayertz 2005; Fukuyama 2004; Kettner 2006; Krüger 2004, 2010).

During approximately the same period, the amount of care provided at home by the family decreased due to, among other things, women increasingly working outside the home, changes in the traditional family structure, and the greater distances between the places in which the various members of the family live (Gronemeyer, M. 2005). The resulting lack of informal or familial care was gradually filled by professional caregiving facilities (Böhm et al 2009: 74; Robert Koch Institut 2004: 51f.), promoting the hospitalization and professionalization of dealing with critically ill and dying patients.

---

3   On the connection between the definition of brain death and organ transplants, see also Müller (2010).

"FEAR OF HIGH TECH MEDICINE"—
A DRIVING FORCE FOR DISCOURSE

A key feature of the death debates in recent years has been that they linked the issue of medical technology and its social status to an allegedly widespread fear of prolonging life "at all costs". These two very different things are widely discussed in a way that suggests a causal connection: a large share of the population, allegedly, is afraid of being kept alive only with the aid of "high-tech medicine". It is not clear whether and to which extent this fear is indeed present among the population, but it certainly is very prominent in public discourse. To avoid this situation and to sooth public fears, so the story goes, we need legal means to limit medical treatment at the end of life. That way, the imagined problems of imagined incapacitated patients in public discourse fuel the demand for freedom of choice and patient autonomy—interpreted as "making decisions for oneself".

An image circulating throughout the debates, conveying a specific perspective on dying is that of a person whose life is dependent on a machine.[4] What this image connotes is that people are afraid and also have to be afraid of "being attached to a machine," incapable of making a choice, and being dependent on the actions of caregivers and doctors. It is closely linked to the discourse on "prolonging life at all costs".[5] In this way, the

---

[4] If one looks for the origin of this image, one comes across the notion transported by the attempt to manufacture an artificial heart and the heart-lung apparatus: the first images shown in the media were featuring a "person attached to a machine" whose operation was dependent on an electric socket! (Thoms 2009)

[5] Interestingly enough, the Recommendations by the German Medical Association and the Central Ethics Commission at the German Medical Association on Dealing with Health Care Powers of Attorney and Living Wills in Medical Practice make reference to "high-tech medicine" as well: "By providing the patient with as detailed information as possible, the physician can at the same time take precautions against patient provisions not required from a medical point of view, for example by clearing up misunderstandings—e.g., about so-called high-tech medicine—correcting false estimations with respect to the kind and statistical distribution of the courses of disease, and questioning the experience had in the patient's environment toward which he or she orients him- or herself and from which he or she possibly makes false conclusions" (Bundesärztekammer 2010).

discourse is supported and kept alive by an assumed but unresolved concept. Thus, in public discourse, criticism of mechanization in medicine in the past few years has led directly to the demand for "self-determination at the end of life"—exercised through limiting therapy. High technology in medicine has thus become a "linchpin" in the public debates on active euthanasia, limitation of terminal care, and the binding character of the living will.

According to the philosopher, Catholic priest, and medicine critic Ivan Illich, a medicalization of dying has occurred in recent decades (Illich 1995), that entails among other things that other "benevolent" kinds of assistance during dying are neglected. Although dying at home can be accompanied by outpatient care, today many people feel overwhelmed by caring for dying family members at home. For one thing, this care is made difficult or even impossible by the fact that many people work outside the home and extended families no longer live under one roof, and, for another, "embedding dying in professional care results in the family being compelled to regard itself as not responsible" (Gronemeyer, R. 1995: 211). One reason for the exploding discourse on how and when people die may therefore be the fact that more and more people die in clinical institutions in which they are professionally treated with the aid of medical technology. In addition, dying people are viewed as "patients" that require medical treatment. Thus, dying is no longer considered the final phase of a person's life, but rather as a state in which medical intervention is necessary.

Unspectacular, somehow natural dying has today turned into medically controlled dying that for the most part occurs in a hospital or a nursing home: 80 percent of all Germans die in an institution, although 80% of all Germans state that they would like to die at home. (Gronemeyer 2007: 16)

In the debates on dying, the assumption that a major share of the population fears being kept alive by means of "high-tech medicine" and against one's will becomes an argument for legalizing active physician-assisted euthanasia, extended hospice and palliative care, and the binding force of a living will and, if necessary, a representative in form of a guardian or an authorized person in health-related matters. In the following, I will discuss these links on the basis of documents that are part of the debates on dying.

Living Will and Active Euthanasia

A debate has taken place in Germany on the legalization of active euthanasia since the 1960s. Since the early 1980s it has led to the founding of euthanasia associations. This debate mainly features the concepts of self-determination and patient autonomy. According to the *Deutsche Gesellschaft für Humanes Sterben* (German Society for Dying in Dignity, DGHS), the discussion surrounding living wills in Germany was taken up in the 1970s (Deutsche Gesellschaft für Humanes Sterben 2006: 50). The DGHS has demanded the chance of exercising self-determination with the aid of a living will for years. Accordingly, they welcomed the fulfillment of this demand in September 2009 through the enactment of the Third Statute for the Revision of the Guardianship Law (Neumann 2007; Deutsche Gesellschaft für Humanes Sterben 2006, 2010).

Up to recent years, the so-called euthanasia associations in Germany had a difficulty standing. The experience of the National Socialist "euthanasia" program was, and remains, a daunting memory in large parts of the population, politics, and the medical community (Wunder 2000: 251). Advances in the direction of "voluntary euthanasia" and "active euthanasia" continue to be perceived as "offensive," yet they are also heatedly discussed. This is reflected, for example, in the results of an anonymous survey of physicians' attitudes on active euthanasia and physician-assisted dying (Anonyme Umfrage 2008) or on the Web site *pro sterbehilfe*, set up by doctors in 2007, where one can sign an appeal for physician-assisted dying (Arnold 2007). In recent years, an open discussion is taking place among the public as well as within the medical or the bioethics community and many voices argue that under certain circumstances, the absolute prohibition of assisted dying should be abandoned (see Birnbacher 2004; Minelli 2007; Hoerster 1998, 2007; Putz 2007). The opening of an office by the Swiss assisted dying association Dignitas 2005 in Hanover showed how quickly a debate on "assisted suicide" can enter the political agenda, although in Germany, the administration of substances that cause death is prohibited under the *Arzneimittelgesetz* (German Pharmaceuticals Act).[6]

---

6   The German Pharmaceuticals Act regulates the marketing of pharmaceuticals and seeks to ensure an "adequate supply of pharmaceuticals to human beings and animals, safety in the marketing of pharmaceuticals," and provide "in par-

Since 1980, the DGHS's campaign for the legalization of active euthanasia has been generating a great deal of media attention:

The German Society for Dying in Dignity (DGHS) advocates sparing people from intolerable and senseless suffering and maintaining their human dignity even while dying. It seeks to improve the conditions for the terminally ill and dying in this country. (Deutsche Gesellschaft für Humanes Sterben 2010)

The association views self-determination at the end of one's life as a human and civil right that includes the "right to reduce the duration of death for humanitarian reasons" (Deutsche Gesellschaft für Humanes Sterben 2010).

In its Guideline(s) with Respect to Legal Policy on Living Wills and Assisted Euthanasia from 2004, the association addresses people who agree that "the will of the patient concerned" be given "more weight in day-to-day care and dying" and who are "dissatisfied with the existing legal situation in Germany." The DGHS assumes that there are a large number of people who believe that those who are elderly, terminally ill, or require care in Germany need both, "more care and more freedom." They therefore think that "the promotion of autonomy and self-determination should be equally as important as the promotion of palliative medicine and terminal care". They "suspect that palliative medicine in no way makes all demands for physician-assisted suicide and active, direct euthanasia superfluous." (Deutsche Gesellschaft für Humanes Sterben 2010).

The association contends that many people "are unwilling to let others dictate how they are to die" and vehemently opposes the prevailing "blockade mentality in political, church, and professional medical circles" (Deutsche Gesellschaft für Humanes Sterben 2010). It calls for "clear, appropriately objective, and comprehensive guidelines regarding assisted death in criminal and civil law". Their goals is a legal framework for assisted death in order to

assert the right of all individuals suffering from terminal illness to make the ultimate decision about their own life and death and to dictate the type and scope of medical procedures to be carried out and whether they are to be continued or discontinued, to

---

ticular for the quality, efficacy, and reliability of pharmaceuticals" (Arzneimittelgesetz 1976).

the extent their condition permits" (Deutsche Gesellschaft für Humanes Sterben 2010).

According to the association, the patient's right to self-determination must be strengthened in general, even in cases in which continued treatment is indicated from a medical point of view.

The patient's right of self-determination takes precedence over the physician's desire to help. This holds true even when the patient rejects a measure or has previously rejected an anticipated measure which is certainly or probably in his or her own interest or when the measure in question involves artificial respiration, the administration of fluids, or artificial nutrition. The right of self-determination also encompasses the right to life-sustaining treatment within medically reasonable limits. (Deutsche Gesellschaft für Humanes Sterben 2010)

The association adds:

The statutory guidelines should definitively establish the legality of discontinuing or failing to initiate life-sustaining measures in response to a patient's express wish and intent, or when a patient has previously expressed such a wish and intent in anticipation, or when a patient is permanently incapable of declaring such a wish or intent and reliable indications support the assumption that he or she would reject the treatment in question. The determining factor should be the patient's express or presumed wish and not his or her well-being—as assessed from the perspective of another person. (Deutsche Gesellschaft für Humanes Sterben 2010)

The phrase "expressed previously in anticipation" as applied to patients' wishes points to the instrument of the living will, as is clearly indicated in the following paragraph: the option of "prolonging treatment or reverting to palliative measures" must also be available to patients who are capable of giving consent (Deutsche Gesellschaft für Humanes Sterben 2010). But what if a patient is not capable of expressing consent? The DGHS' answer to this question is:

In order to respond appropriately to the needs of patients who are incapable of expressing consent, the living will should be firmly established in guardianship law. The key element of the guidelines adopted by the German Medical Association with respect to medical assistance for the dying could serve as a guiding principle: A living will is binding in so far as it pertains to a specific treatment situation and no circumstances are evident that would indicate that the patient no longer wishes it to apply. (Deutsche Gesellschaft für Humanes Sterben 2010)

It is interesting to note that this demand expressed by the DGHS has been incorporated precisely into the Third Statute for the Revision of the Guardianship Law of July 29, 2009. Article 1, Section 1901a (1) of this law states the following:

If an adult capable of expressing consent has specified in writing that, in the event that he or she should be incapable of giving consent, he or she consents to or rejects specific medical examinations, medical treatment, or medical procedures which are not immediately indicated at the time at which they are specified (living will), the guardian shall determine whether these specifications apply to the patient's current health and treatment situation. If so, the guardian is obliged to voice the patient's wishes and ensure that they are carried out. (Drittes Gesetz zur Änderung des Betreuungsrechts 2009)

However, the DGHS also calls for binding rules for less clearly defined situations:

Living wills should also be regarded as binding in situations for which they have not been expressly written but to which they may reasonably be applied and in which there can be no doubt that the patient would have intended them to apply. Living wills should be regarded by physicians as well as courts, guardians, and authorized representatives as expressions of a patient's earlier wishes. Guardianship law should clearly provide that decisions by guardians and authorized representatives must reflect the express wishes of the patient or, if no explicit declaration of wishes is available, the presumed wishes of the patient and his or her purely personal concept of human dignity. (Deutsche Gesellschaft für Humanes Sterben 2010)

This demand has also been adopted by the Third Statute for the Revision of the Guardianship Law, which specifies as follows in Section 2:

In the absence of a living will or in cases in which the instructions contained in a living will do not apply to a patient's present health and treatment situation, the guardian is obliged to identify the patient's actual or presumed wishes regarding treatment and decide on that basis whether to consent to or reject a medical procedure in accordance with Section 1. The patient's presumed wishes are to be determined with reference to specific indicators. Indicators to be considered include in particular previous oral or written statements, ethical or religious convictions, and other personal values embraced by the patient. (Drittes Gesetz zur Änderung des Betreuungsrechts 2009)

The DGHS also advocates the adoption of new laws regarding active euthanasia.

Direct active euthanasia, i.e., euthanasia undertaken for the purpose of putting an end to suffering, in which the act is not controlled by the terminally ill patient but by another individual, should be permitted by law in rare, extreme cases only, according to the DGHS. This restriction is necessary in order to prevent the risks of abuse, loss of trust, and the extension of active euthanasia to include cases of sympathy killing in which the terminally ill patient does not or has not expressed the wish to die. (Deutsche Gesellschaft für Humanes Sterben 2010)

Thus, they argue, an exemption from legal sanctions should be possible in extreme cases when a terminally ill patient who wishes to die but "is not physically capable of committing suicide" is put to death by another person. In this context, the DGHS refers to an addendum to Section 216 of the German Criminal Code proposed in 1985 by the authors of the *Alternativentwurf eines Gesetzes über Sterbehilfe—AE Sterbehilfe* (Alternative Draft of a Law on Active Euthanasia—AE Active Euthanasia) (Bauman et al 1986). The AE Active Euthanasia retains the principle that active euthanasia should remain illegal except in cases in which specific, clearly defined criteria apply. In the opinion of the DGHS, such a solution is unacceptable. The association proposes that the situation described should not be interpreted as killing on demand, as it is regarded as morally different by the association.

Active euthanasia performed under the restricted conditions described is regarded in our society as morally acceptable and perhaps even morally necessary. The idea that exemption from punishment should be elective only is also unacceptable, as it still exposes the acting physician to the risk of punishment under criminal law. The

DGHS demands instead that exemption from legal sanctions be defined as the rule, rather than the exception, under the conditions defined. (Deutsche Gesellschaft für Humanes Sterben 2010)

The DGHS advocates self-determination or patient autonomy. At the same time, the association also calls for the legalization of active euthanasia performed in "rare, extreme cases." The option of deciding to be put to death with the assistance of a physician under certain circumstances is regarded by the association as an individual right of self-determination. The DGHS has expressed great satisfaction with progress on the issue of living wills and provides extensive material on the subject at its homepage (Deutsche Gesellschaft für Humanes Sterben 2010). The association sees one of its most important demands achieved in the *Patienten-Schutz-Gesetz* (Patient Rights Act) which took effect on September 1, 2009, a demand to which it has been consistently committed since its founding. That commitment is documented in numerous campaigns and publications, including a position paper on the ethics of death, which was approved for release by the DGHS General Membership Meeting on November 27, 2008 (Deutsche Gesellschaft für Humanes Sterben 2008).

The statements issued by the DGHS clearly indicate how arguments in support of patient autonomy (advanced within the context of the debate on living wills) lead to the demand for socially regulated active, physician-assisted euthanasia. Concern with the issues associated with a paternalistic physician-patient relationship culminate in the demand to strengthen patients' rights to the extent that, expressed at a given time or articulated by a currently unconscious patient in a previous living will, a patient's wishes must take precedence over medical indications. Through the instrument of the living will, patient autonomy must be recognized as absolute, even in—exceptional—cases involving the issue of active, physician-assisted euthanasia.

LIVING WILLS AND HOSPICE OR PALLIATIVE CARE

The modern hospice movement that arose in the late 1960s represented a counterweight to the recurring debate on "terminal care." Palliative medicine, which had emerged from a medical context in the 1980s, was oriented toward concepts of care developed by the hospice movement (Godzik 1992). Both approaches to care for the dying—palliative medicine and the hospice movement—reflect the need to relieve pain and suffering and the urgency of the appeal for a care concept that responds to the specific needs of severely ill and dying patients. Both are opposed to active euthanasia.

However, practitioners of hospice care and palliative medicine also advocate self-determination in dying, and seek to offer terminally ill patients an opportunity to take control of their individual death processes in the sense of choosing a "personal" way of dying. Both the hospice movement and palliative medicine recognize the role of the living will in their efforts to deal with death and dying.

In 2005, the former *Bundesarbeitsgemeinschaft Hospiz*, which has since been renamed as the *Deutscher Hospiz und PalliativVerband* (German Hospice and Palliative Care Association), issued a number of recommendations on the subject of living wills. Its summary findings (Sabatowski et al 2005: 2) are based on rules and procedures which must be faithfully observed. The authors of these summary findings conclude that experience in the field of hospice care has shown that care for the dying requires a considerable amount of communication. That also applies to the process of drafting a living will, which involves not only the written expression of a patient's wishes but also a communication process through which those wishes take form. The framework that gives strength and stability to a living will is built in the course of discussions with relatives, physicians, and others.

Only the active effort to come to terms with one's own life will make it possible to shape the process of dying in such a way that both life and death reflect one's own wishes. Through interaction, family doctors and people close to the patient acquire a foundation that enables them to identify the patient's presumed wishes. (Sabatowski et al 2005: 2)

Sabatowski and other proponents of living wills regard them as an essential aspect of hospice care. How best to invite people to approach the subject of a living will? Evidently, they argue, it is best approached through a "communication process." Being invited to talk about one's own death is a prerequisite for the conception and preparation of a living will, thus communication, they suggest, is a good starting point. The law may form one means to stimulate such communication processes, as the German Hospice and Palliative Care Association argues with regard to the Revision of the Guardianship Law in 2009 in a press release: "Dealing with one's own mortality can be very difficult. The new law provides impulses for the attempt to come to terms with death and dying" (Deutscher Hospiz- und PalliativVerband 2009a: 2). The authors of the press release point out that the law

strengthens the patient's right of self-determination—in a situation in which he or she is no longer capable of making a decision. For the written expression of a patient's wishes regarding treatment or the refusal of treatment for an illness or following an accident assumes a strong binding character on the basis of this law (Deutscher Hospiz- und PalliativVerband 2009a: 1).

The authors also point out the importance of supplementing a living will with a power of attorney specifying which relatives or other individuals are to ensure that the wishes of the patient are carried out (Deutscher Hospiz- und PalliativVerband 2009a: 1).

On August 28, 2009, the Association issued a handout on the new law regarding the living will and its implementation, drafted primarily by attorney Thomas Klie. The document contains the following statement:

The patient's wishes have absolute priority. The legislature regards living wills as fulfilling an important role in ensuring the self-determination of patients at the end of their lives. Neither physicians nor relatives nor guardians have the right to ignore the patient's express wishes. (Deutscher Hospiz- und PalliativVerband 2009b: 1)

This applies to current expressions of will and to written declarations, insofar as they "pertain to specific treatments or medical procedures and are relevant to the patient's current health and treatment situation." Klie goes on to define the nature of the situation in which a written living will is regarded as valid and binding:

Living wills offer the occasion and opportunity for discussion of issues relating to the end of one's life that are often put aside, neglected, or regarded as taboo. Regardless of whether a living will is signed or not, the effort made to come to terms with one's own thoughts, fears, and wishes is worthwhile. The process of drafting a living will is also important, as it provides an occasion for discussing these significant issues relating to the final phase of life with a doctor and with one's partner and relatives. (Deutscher Hospiz- und PalliativVerband 2009b: 3)

The living will takes on additional significance in that it becomes an occasion for personal reflection on aspects of dying and for clarification of one's own thoughts about the circumstances under which one wishes to die in dialogue with relatives, physicians, etc.

The law regarding living wills also offers physicians and nursing personnel in hospitals as well as employees of nursing homes and home nursing services an opportunity to reassess their own approaches to dealing with difficult issues encountered during the final phase of life within their own institutions and professions and to reflect on their ethical and legal ramifications. (Deutscher Hospiz- und PalliativVerband 2009b: 3)

Thus some of those involved in the hospice movement recognize the relevance of the instrument of the living will even though its implementation is the focus of criticism. In the concluding remarks in the handout on the new law regarding living wills and their implementation, however, Klie emphasizes that the instrument of the living will must not tempt one to believe that it can "resolve all of the medical issues" that may arise during the final phase of life.

It is impossible to answer every question in advance. We must realize that our thoughts, feelings and views of the world as well as circumstances and treatment methods can always change. . . . And we must not lose sight of the fact that living wills can be misused, and that others may have a personal interest in having the patient draft such a document. (Deutscher Hospiz- und PalliativVerband 2009b: 12)

However, there as also been criticism of living wills within the hospice and palliative care movement. In an interview published by the *Hospiz-Zeitschrift* in 2000, social psychiatrist Klaus Dörner wrote that that idea of the living will conflicts with the concept of hospice care:

The living will could be harmful in two ways: It could be harmful to me because I do not want to influence this natural uncertainty during the final phase of my life as I approach death through abstract, rational considerations. I want to experience it and, in fact, to suffer through it as it comes. And if I write such a living will for myself, it will also have an effect on caregivers—in hospital intensive care or home hospice care—in that they are concerned only with protecting themselves in the face of the wishes and demands expressed by patients and are thus incapable of performing spontaneous acts required in order to provide care for the dying in an atmosphere of trust. In other words, the living will undermines the concept of hospice care. (Dörner 2000: 9)

Speaking in the culture program *Glaubenssachen* (matters of faith) of *Norddeutscher Rundfunk*, Oliver Tolmein, an author and attorney specialized in medical law who represents numerous disabled clients, points out that:

Self-determined dying is a generally recognized goal; yet, regardless of whether we are capable of making decisions about our own medical treatment during this final phase ourselves or are no longer able to communicate in this form, self-determined dying is an illusion, for what brings us to the point of preparing for our own death is ordinarily beyond our control. Cancer, stroke, dementia, but also gradual physical decline or organ failure are not things for which we would have consciously wished. (Tolmein 2010: 2)

Tolmein points out that the illusion of being able to dictate the medical circumstances of our deaths also has social implications:

It is also a phase in which we need care, in which we depend upon people close to us who will talk to us, encourage us, or enable us to talk about our despair and disappointment—thus, it is a phase of life in which we are more dependent on others than ever (Tolmein 2010: 2).

In later interviews, Tolmein speaks of a cultural shift of values that results from the strengthened right of self-determination:

Human life is made more amenable to disposition. Social responsibility for an individual is forced into the background. Weak people who often need a great deal of help are no longer guaranteed comfort, security, and care. What they get, whether they want it and can use it or not, is a license for self-determination which leaves them to their own devices and robs them of the support they would normally have received from the community as a matter of course. (Tolmein 2010: 3)

The journal of the Medical Association also published a critical article on the subject of living wills in which the German Protestant Church complained that the new law places "one-sided emphasis on patient self-determination," making it impossible to maintain the "balance between self-determination and care" (Deutsches Ärzteblatt 2009).

One of the main focuses of criticism of living wills relates to the inadequate right to counseling. Some critics have even advocated mandatory counseling. Counseling is urgently needed, according to the authors of several recent publications on medical law and ethics (see Vetter/Marckmann 2009; Borasio 2007).

But what do the institutions that provide counseling on living wills actually offer? Informative materials and documents containing recommendations regarding the issue of the living will often begin with an appeal to readers to think about the circumstances of their own deaths. In her foreword to the brochure entitled *Patientenverfügung. Wie bestimme ich, was medizinisch unternommen werden soll, wenn ich entscheidungsunfähig bin?* (The living will: How do I specify what medical procedures will be taken when I am unable to make decisions for myself?), then Federal Minister of Justice Brigitte Zypries discussed the option of expressing one's wishes in a living will, emphasizing that those who do so can now be certain that their wills will be accepted as legally binding in the event that they lose consciousness.

With the Third Statute for the Revision of the Guardianship Law, the living will is now firmly anchored in guardianship law. At last, private citizens as well as physicians, guardians, and others empowered to act on their behalf now have clear legal definitions and more legal certainty with respect to living wills. The law clearly states that people have the right to decide whether and how they wish to be treated during every phase of their life. It also ensures that courts will be authorized to make final decisions in cases involving the danger of misuse or doubts with regard to a patient's wishes. (Bundesministerium für Justiz 2010)

Readers are then asked to think very carefully about the kinds of treatment they wish or do not wish to receive.[7] They are advised to imagine the situations that may arise during the final phase of life in order to decide in advance how they wish to be treated in those situations at a future point in time.

Take the time to consider these difficult matters yourself and to discuss any questions that occur to you with your family doctor or people who work in the relevant organizations. This brochure is meant to encourage you to take timely steps in preparation for the final phase of your life and to provide support in your efforts to do so. (Bundesministerium für Justiz 2010)

The brochure seeks to encourage readers to consider these matters, to imagine future situations, to think ahead, to talk about them, to ask questions, and to make "preparations." In this way, it advises people to imagine their dying circumstances, to think about them, to talk about them with people who are qualified to offer guidance, and to plan their own deaths through this communication process.

At this point, a link is also established to the existing assumption within the debate on death and dying cited above that certain segments of the population are (quite rightly!) afraid of high-tech medicine.

Thanks to scientific and technical progress, we are now able to help severely ill patients who could not possibly have been saved fifty years ago. While this perspective offers hope and opportunities for many people, others are afraid of prolonging their suffering and death with the aid of high-tech medicine. (Bundesministerium für Justiz 2010)

---

7   It is interesting to note that the discourse on death and dying always focuses on the rejection of specific medical procedures. Criticism of the kind expressed by Hubert Hüppe, a Christian Democrat member of the German Bundestag is rare: "But many of the fears regarding high-tech medicine incited in the public no longer have anything to do with reality. On the contrary, it is actually more likely that patients do not receive treatment that is necessary from a medical point of view" (Hüppe 2010).

The newsletter issued by the *Bundeszentralstelle Patientenverfügung* (Federal Office for Living Wills) of the Humanist Society also contains an appeal to readers to consider their own dying process and addresses the assumption of a "fear of high-tech medicine:" "Many people are plagued by the fear of being 'hooked up to a machine' during the final phase of life, helpless and with no prospect of a life that is worth living" (Humanistischer Verband Deutschland 2009).

Thus the Humanist Society advises people to complete their living wills and offers corresponding guidance and instructions. Since October 2009, the association has been distributing a so-called Standard Living Will bearing the subtitle ... *wenn es medizinisch aussichtslos ist* (... when medicine no longer offers hope). The document contains text modules drafted by the Federal Ministry of Justice, a practical "check-the-box" form, "expert advice," and a "power of attorney for guardians" (Humanistischer Verband Deutschland 2009). Those who are interested can also order a brochure entitled *Optimale Patientenverfügung* (The Ideal Living Will) containing a questionnaire to be used in preparing a "qualified ideal living will." The questionnaire contains questions about a person's current health; attitudes about death and dying; views regarding intensive medicine, emergency rescue measures, and reanimation; about "quality of life in cases of permanent physical disability and suffering;" about hopes in the event of brain injury, coma, long-term waking coma; and opinions regarding dignity, progressive mental impairment and dementia, pain therapy, palliative medicine, statements about how and where a person wishes to die, advance powers of attorney, and attitudes about artificial nutrition (Humanistischer Verband Deutschland 2009).

The underlying objective is to encourage people to imagine themselves in a variety of conceivable situations which could arise during the final phase of life and to make preparations and arrangements for these potential future situations—today. This option to decide is coupled with a perceived fear—which is also attributed to segments of the population—of being controlled by a medical apparatus designed to prolong life or even the process of dying.

THE LIVING WILL AS A PLANNING INSTRUMENT FOR THE PROCESS OF DYING

What is going on here? What is the purpose of the frequently discussed living will? Its objective is the design, indeed the planning of the last phase of life, the process of dying. I suggest that the living will can be regarded as a set of rules which unites the demands expressed by different groups with regard to the treatment of those who are dying. Patient autonomy, these groups argue, is to be given a legally binding form of expression. At the same time, attending physicians and caregivers as well as relatives are to be relieved of the responsibility of making the right decision in the patient's interest. Self-determination, in this view, should not only be practically amenable to planning but also anchored in law and accessible to every individual. Thus, we can understand the living will as a set of rules which invites, if not obliges, an individual to plan the circumstances of his or her death and to specify the binding character of this plan even in cases he or she is unconscious or otherwise is incapable of expressing his or her wishes.

There is now evidence of near-unanimous agreement in German public discourse that the living will is an instrument which can foster self-determination of people who are dying as well as those who are not faced with impending death. This is somewhat confusing in view of the circumstances cited at the beginning of this paper. Up to now, the advocates and opponents of active euthanasia have occupied two opposing fronts in the debate on death and dying. The common focus on self-determination through the instrument of the living will has now made it possible for these two formerly antagonistic positions to converge.

The debates on dying convey the appeal to plan the medical circumstances of one's own dying process and to make appropriate preparations for every conceivable death-bed situation. This is achieved through the expression of a need—the need for someone to make a decision in a situation in which an individual must be given life-prolonging treatment, for example, because he or she cannot survive without long-term medical-technical assistance in the form of artificial respiration or nutrition. And because such decisions must be—and inevitably are—made, it is best that they be made by the individuals themselves.

The instrument of the living will provides a platform on which people with differing views regarding the treatment of the dying can come together, even though the implementation of living wills is still a focus of criticism from some corners. The development of the living will is welcomed by associations concerned with the subject of assisted dying, such as the DGHS, and it is coupled with yet another political demand: the demand to legalize active euthanasia. The instrument of the living will is accepted by at least parts of the hospice movement and some palliative care institutions, although one occasionally has the impression that these circles are concerned primarily with the issue because it is a current, politically relevant topic within the debate on death and dying that has been addressed within the context of the discourse on hospice care, although it really has no place there.

Such a convergence is understandable in light of the importance attached to the concept of patient autonomy. Today, there is broad consensus in support of measures to strengthen patient autonomy and—particularly in conflict situations during the final phase of life—preventing the development of a paternalistic physician-patient relationship.

It is entirely conceivable that some people will be unwilling to concern themselves with medical issues at all as they approach the end of their life, at least not in the sense of imagining their own death, anticipating situations that could arise during the final phase of life, or being forced to make decisions about medical treatment during their dying days. It is quite possible that some people even regard this as an unreasonable expectation and prefer to depend on friends and relatives and to trust them to do what is right. No one has to draft a living will: "Of course no one is obligated to write a living will," according to the informative brochure on living wills issued by the Federal Ministry of Justice (Bundesministerium der Justiz 2010: 10). Yet the debate conveys the sense that it is necessary to think about the process of dying, as otherwise decisions will be taken out of my hands. Reflecting on the important and highly personal subject of dying, imagining it, discussing it, consulting with experts about it, instructing others on how to act as I approach death—these activities are governed by a certain structure. I transpose my thoughts regarding my own death into a procedural structure, a communication process that should culminate in a decision: the decision-making option I can and must choose because it is recognized by society, because it has become a matter of social consensus, because the opportunity exists and should be seized. Through the communication process, my dying becomes a process that can be planned.

The act of talking about dying is institutionalized in the debates on death and dying. People are called upon to think about, discuss, and make decisions about the circumstances under which they wish to die. Yet these decisions are guided by the format of living wills and restricted to certain narrow limits. People are now expected to anticipate, make decisions upon and plan their own death. Thus the option to just say: "I am placing my death in your hands. I am relying on you to do what is right" is no longer available. If I rejected the option to set up a living will other would consider me naïve, if not irresponsible. I would be acting irresponsibly insofar as I would fail to exercise self-determination; instead I would burden others with the responsibility of making decisions that concern me, and quite possibly ask too much of them in doing so.

In the debates on dying, my own dying is viewed as a problem that is approached and "solved" through a standardized process of communication and thus leads to the social management of death and dying. The procedural form forces me to equate two different spheres: I am supposed to imagine terminal situations that can currently occur and specify a—possible!—future medical response. The appeal to plan the dying process is presented as a matter of self-determination, as an option to decide.

The discourses on self-determined planning or design of the dying process suggests that it is necessary to plan ahead at a time when one is still "in command of one's faculties" in order to prepare for a situation in which one is powerless, for example, by drafting a living will or by requesting active euthanasia. This results in an individualization of the process of dying; people are expected to plan their own dying process because it is assumed for a fact that they cannot rely on others when they are most vulnerable. My trust in my relatives and others around me, my faith that they will do what is right and that I can feel cared for humanly, diminishes and may even disappear. They give way to the norm of making decisions about how I wish to die, of planning and arranging for my own death. The guiding ethical principle of patient autonomy is strongly supported by the instrument of the living will. On the other hand, responsible or caring actions on behalf of the patient play an increasingly minor role. A tendency may emerge in which self-determined action in medical situations during the final phase of life gradually becomes a social norm, something that is expected of the patient, while the obligation to care for those who are ill—once firmly anchored in medical ethics—fades into the background.

Translation by Rebecca van Dyck

REFERENCES

Aries, Phillippe (1995): Geschichte des Todes, Munich: Deutscher Taschenbuch.
Arnold, Uwe-Christian (2007): Solidaritätsaufruf Sterbehilfe, available at http//:www.prosterbehilfe.de (last accessed 10/5/2010).
Anonyme Umfrage (2008): Anonyme Ärzteumfrage zu aktiver Sterbehilfe und ärztlicher Suizidbeihilfe, available at http://www.spiegel.de/politik/debatte/de (last accessed 4/30/2010).
Bauer, Axel W. (2006): "Autonomie am Lebensende: Realität, Ideal, Illusion?", in: Universitas 61, Nr. 716, Stuttgart: S. Hirtzel , pp. 115-131.
Baumann, Jürgen/Bochnik, Hans Joachim/Brauneck, Anne-Eva/Calliess, Rolf-Peter et al (eds) (1986): Alternativentwurf eines Gesetzes über Sterbehilfe (AE-Sterbehilfe), Stuttgart: Thieme.
Bayertz, Kurt (ed) (2005): Die menschliche Natur: welchen und wieviel Wert hat sie? Paderborn: Mentis.
Birnbacher, Dieter (2004): "Terminale Sedierung, Sterbehilfe und kausale Rollen", in: Ethik in der Medizin 16, Heft 4, pp. 358-368.
Böhm, Karin/Tesch-Römer, Clemens/Ziese, Thomas (ed) (2009): Beiträge zur Gesundheitsberichterstattung des Bundes, Schwerpunktbericht: Pflege. Gesundheit und Krankheit im Alter, Berlin: Statistisches Bundesamt.
Borasio, Gian Domenico/Heßler, Hans-Joachim/Wiesing, Urban (2009): "Patientenverfügungsgesetz: Umsetzung in der klinischen Praxis", in: Deutsches Ärzteblatt; 106(40): A-1952 / B-1675 / C-1643.
Bundesärztekammer (2010): "Empfehlungen der Bundesärztekammer und der Zentralen Ethikkommission bei der Bundesärztekammer zum Umgang mit Vorsorgevollmacht und Patientenverfügung in der ärztlichen Praxis", in: Deutsches Ärzteblatt, 107(18): A-877 / B- 769 / C-757.
Bundesministerium für Justiz (1976): Gesetz über den Verkehr mit Arzneimitteln (Arzneimittelgesetz AMG).

Bundesministerium für Justiz (2010): Leiden - Krankheit - Sterben: Wie bestimme ich, was medizinisch unternommen werden soll, wenn ich entscheidungsunfähig bin? available at http://www.bmj.bund.de/Publi kationen/Patientenverfuegung_oe.html (last accessed 4/14/2010).

Bundesgerichtshof (2003): XII. Zivilsenat: Beschluss vom 17. März 2003, Aktenzeichen XII ZB 2/03.

Charbonnier, Ralph/May, Anrdt T./Neitzke, Gerald (2005): "Patientenverfügungen in der öffentlichen Diskussion", in: May, Arnd T./Charbonnier, Ralph (eds) (2005): Patientenverfügungen. Unterschiedliche Regelungsmöglichkeiten zwischen Selbstbestimmung und Fürsorge, Münster: LIT, pp. 9-13.

Deutsches Ärzteblatt (2009): "Patientenverfügungsgesetz: Kritik von Kirchen und Hospiz-Stiftung", 6/19/2009, available at http://www.aerzte blatt.de/v4/news/news.asp?id=37020&src=suche&p=patientenverf%FC gung+kirche (last accessed 8/30/2010).

Deutsche Gesellschaft für Humanes Sterben (2006): "Die Anfänge der Patientenverfügungen in Deutschland. Wie sich die Idee der Selbstbestimmung am Lebensende etwa ab Mitte der 70er Jahre allmählich bei uns verbreitete", in: Humanes Leben – Humanes Sterben 4/2006.

— (2008): Positionspapier, 11/27/2008, available at http://www.dghs.de (last accessed 3/30/2010).

— (2010): Homepage der Deutschen Gesellschaft für Humanes Sterben, Selbstverständnis und Grundsatz-Positionen, available at http://www. dghs.de (last accessed 3/30/2010).

Deutsche Hospiz Stiftung (2008): Hospizliche Begleitung und Palliative-Care-Versorgung in Deutschland 2007 (2/26/2008).

Deutscher Hospiz- und PalliativVerband (2009a): Presseerklärung.

— (2009b): Handreichung zum neuen Gesetz zur Regelung der Patientenverfügung und seiner Umsetzung, maßgeblich erarbeitet von Rechtsanwalt Prof. Dr. Thomas Klie, 8/28/2009.

Dörner, Klaus (2000): "Wer verfügt über das Sterben? Patientenverfügungen", in: Die Hospiz-Zeitschrift 2 (2000), Ausgabe 3, pp. 5-9, available at http://www.pkgodzik.de/Auszug%20Doerner.htm (last accessed 3/ 30/2010).

Drittes Gesetz zur Änderung des Betreuungsrechts (2009): Bundesgesetzblatt Jahrgang 2009 Teil I Nr. 48, ausgegeben zu Bonn am 31. Juli 2009, pp. 2287-2287, available at http://www.bmj.bund.de/files/-/3906/

Drittes_Gesetz_Aenderung_Betreuungsrecht_Bundesgesetzblatt.pdf (last accessed 9/30/2010).

Endreß, Alexander/Bauer, Michael (eds) (2007): Selbstbestimmung am Ende des Lebens, Aschaffenburg: Alibri.

Frewer, Andreas/Eickhoff, Clemens (eds) (2000): "Euthanasie" und die aktuelle Sterbehilfe-Debatte. Die historischen Hintergründe medizinischer Ethik, Frankfurt a.M.: Campus.

Fukuyama, Francis (2004): "Transhumanism", in: Foreign Policy 124, pp. 42-44.

Godzik, Peter (1992): Zur Geschichte der Hospizbewegung in Deutschland, available at http://www.pkgodzik.de/fileadmin/user_upload/Hospizarbeit/Geschichte_der_Hospizarbeit.pdf (last accessed 8/30/2010).

Gronemeyer, Marianne (2005): "Sterbeorte"; Beitrag zur Tagung "Das Sterben in die Mitte holen", 11/11/2005, available at http://www.imew.de/index.php?id=310 (last accessed 4/30/2010).

Gronemeyer, Reimer (2005): "Hospiz, Hospizbewegung und Palliative Care in Europa", in: Knoblauch, Hubert/Arnold Zingerle (eds): Thanatosoziologie. Tod, Hospiz und die Institutionalisierung des Sterbens, Berlin: Dunker & Humblot, pp. 207-217.

— (2007): Sterben in Deutschland. Wie wir dem Tod wieder einen Platz in unserem Leben einräumen können, Frankfurt a.M.: Fischer.

Hoerster, Norbert (1998): Sterbehilfe im säkularen Staat, Frankfurt a.M.: Suhrkamp.

— (2007): "Rechtsethische Überlegungen zur Sterbehilfe", in: Endreß, Alexander/Bauer, Michael (eds) (2007): Selbstbestimmung am Ende des Lebens, Aschaffenburg: Alibri, pp. 37-50.

Humanistischer Verband Deutschland (2009): Optimale Patientenverfügung. Willensstark, Berlin: Eigendruck.

— (2009): Standard-Patientenverfügung. …wenn es medizinisch aussichtslos ist, Berlin: Eigendruck.

Hüppe, Hubert (2010): Interview available at http://www.patientenverfügung.de/print/3977 (last accessed 3/30/2010).

Huxley, Julian (1957): New Bottles for New Wine, London: Chatto & Windus.

Illich, Ivan (1995): Die Nemesis der Medizin. Die Kritik der Medikalisierung des Lebens, Munich: Suhrkamp.

Jordan, Isabella (2007): Hospizbewegung in Deutschland und den Niederlanden. Palliativversorgung und Selbstbestimmung, Frankfurt a.M.: Campus.

Jordan, Isabella/Frewer, Andreas (2008): "Menschliches Sterben im Wandel? Debatten um eine präventive Medikalisierung des Sterbens", in: Schäfer, Daniel/Frewer, Andreas/Schockenhoff, Eberhard/Wetzstein, Verena (eds): Gesundheitskonzepte im Wandel. Geschichte, Ethik und Gesellschaft, Stuttgart: Steiner, pp. 243-277.

Jordan, Isabella/Hilt, Annette/Frewer, Andreas (eds) (2010): Endlichkeit, Medizin und Unsterblichkeit, Stuttgart: Steiner.

Kettner, Matthias (2005): "Transhumanismus und Körperfeindlichkeit", in: Ach J. S./Pollmann, A. (eds): No body is perfect. Baumaßnahmen am menschlichen Körper. Bioethische und ästhetische Aufrisse, Bielefeld: Transcript, pp. 111-131.

— (ed) (2006): "Wunscherfüllende Medizin" [Themenheft], Ethik in der Medizin 18 (1).

Krüger, Oliver (2004): Virtualität und Unsterblichkeit. Die Visionen des Posthumanismus, Freiburg: Rombach.

— (2010): "Der Tote als Patient – kryonische Unsterblichkeitshoffnungen innerhalb des Transhumanismus", in: Hilt, Annette/Jordan, Isabella/Frewer, Andreas (eds): Endlichkeit, Medizin und Unsterblichkeit, Stuttgart: Steiner, pp. 171-190.

Nationaler Ethikrat (ed) (2005): Patientenverfügung. Ein Instrument der Selbstbestimmung, Stellungnahme 6/2/2005, pp. 207-225.

— (2006): Selbstbestimmung und Fürsorge am Lebensende. Stellungnahme, Berlin.

May, Arnd T./Charbonnier, Ralph (eds) (2005): Patientenverfügungen. Unterschiedliche Regelungsmöglichkeiten zwischen Selbstbestimmung und Fürsorge, Münster: LIT.

McNamee, M./Edwards, S. (2006): "Transhumanism, medical technology and slippery slopes", in: Journal of Medical Ethics 32, pp. 513-518.

Meran, Johannes G./Geissendörfer, Sylke E./May, Arnd T./Simon, Alfred (eds) (2002): Möglichkeiten einer standardisierten Patientenverfügung. Gutachten im Auftrag des Bundesministeriums der Gesundheit, Münster: LIT, pp. 59-77.

Minelli, Ludwig A. (2007): "Muss man nach Deutschland Vernunft importieren? Die eigenartigen Wege der Diskussion um Sterbehilfe", in: Endreß, Alexander/Bauer, Michael (eds) (2007): Selbstbestimmung am Ende des Lebens, Aschaffenburg: Alibri, pp. 146-166.

Muggenthaler, F. (2004): "Die Tiefkühlreligion", in: Die Zeit 42, pp. 1-4.

Müller, Sabine (2010): "Revival der Hirntod-Debatte: Funktionelle Bildgebung für die Hirntod-Diagnostik", in: Ethik in der Medizin (2010) Bd. 22, pp. 5-17.

Neumann, Gitta (2007): "Patientenverfügungen als Instrument der Selbstbestimmung am Ende des Lebens", in: Endreß, Alexander/Bauer, Michael (eds) (2007): Selbstbestimmung am Ende des Lebens, Aschaffenburg: Alibri, pp. 137-145.

Oduncu, Fuat (ed) (1998): Hirntod und Organtransplantation. Medizinische, juristische und ethische Fragen. Göttingen: Vandenhoeck & Ruprecht.

Putz, Wolfgang (2007): "Patientenautonomie im Gerichtssaal", in: Endreß, Alexander/Bauer, Michael (eds) (2007): Selbstbestimmung am Ende des Lebens, Aschaffenburg: Alibri, pp. 27-36.

Robert Koch Institut (2004): Gesundheitsberichterstattung des Bundes, Schwerpunktbericht Pflege, Berlin: Statistisches Bundesamt.

Sabatowski, Rainer/Radbruch, Lukas/Nauck, Roß, F./Zernikow, Boris (2005): Wegweiser Hospiz und Palliativmedizin Deutschland, Wuppertal: Hospiz, p. 2.

Sahm, Stephan (2006): Sterbebegleitung und Patientenverfügung. Ärztliches Handeln an den Grenzen von Ethik und Recht, Frankfurt a.M.: Campus.

Schlich, Thomas/Wiesemann, Claudia (eds) (2001): Hirntod. Zur Kulturgeschichte der Todesfeststellung, Frankfurt a.M.: Suhrkamp.

Statistisches Bundesamt (2010): Destatis. VIII A Gesundheitswesen: Gestorbene insgesamt und in Krankenhäusern 1953-2008.

Student, Christoph (2009): Zu Hause sterben. Hilfen für Betroffene und Angehörige, available at http://christoph-student.homepage.t-online.de/ Zu%20Hause%20sterben%2009.pdf?foo=0.6762176101188486 (last accessed 8/30/2010).

Thoms, Ulrike (2009): "Das umstrittene Experiment: Der Mensch. Biowissenschaftliche Visionen und ihre Realisierung in der BRD der 60er und 70er Jahre", presentation delivered at the DGGMNT conference in September 2009 in Hanover.

Tolmein, Oliver (2010): "Lebensmut und Sterbehilfe. Über Würde, Abschied und Weitermachen"; Hörfunk-Sendung "Glaubenssachen" des Norddeutschen Rundfunks 2/14/2010, Manuskript pp. 1-6.

Vetter, Petra/Marckmann, Georg (2009): "Gesetzliche Regelung der Patientenverfügung: Was ändert sich für die Praxis?", in: Ärzteblatt Baden-Württemberg 64(9), pp. 370-374.

Wehkamp, Karl-Heinz (1998): Sterben und Töten. Euthanasie aus der Sicht deutscher Ärztinnen und Ärzte. Ergebnisse einer empirischen Studie, Berliner Medizinethische Schriften, Heft 23, Berlin.

Wunder, Michael (2000): "Medizin und Gewissen – Die neue Euthanasie-Debatte in Deutschland vor dem historischen und internationalen Hintergrund"; in: Frewer, Andreas/Eickhoff, Clemens (eds): "Euthanasie" und die aktuelle Sterbehilfe-Debatte. Die historischen Hintergründe medizinischer Ethik, Frankfurt a.M.: Campus, pp. 251-275.

Zypries, Brigitte (2007): "Ich will schmerzfrei sterben". Brigitte Zypries über das Recht auf Selbstbestimmung, die Pflicht der Ärzte – und über ihre eigene, persönliche Patientenverfügung. Ein ZEIT-Gespräch mit der Justizministerin, available at http://www.zeit.de/2007/13/Sterben (last accessed 10/8/2010).

Genetic counseling and the fiction of choice: Taught self-determination as a new technique of social engineering[1]

SILJA SAMERSKI

For nearly a century, "self-determination" has been a watchword for women activists struggling against the co-optation of female fertility by the state. In the early 1930s, feminists like Else Kienle called for a woman's right to self-determination over her body and her life when she opposed § 218, the German law that criminalized abortion (Grossmann 1995, 87–92). In the 1970s, self-determination became a central demand as the second wave women's movement rebelled against a paternalistic medical establishment and declared "my body belongs to me."[2] Today, by contrast, women are no longer obliged to fight to make their own decisions; instead, such responsibility is formally imposed upon them. In Western countries, self-determination and autonomy are now on the agenda of doctors, health insurance companies, pharmaceutical companies, geneticists, and research policy makers (Lupton 1995). An increasing number of medical tests and

---

1 First published in Signs, Vol. 34, No. 4.,2009, pp. 735-761, (c) 2009 by The University of Chicago, reprinted by permission of The University of Chicago Press. I thank the anonymous reviewers of Signs for their valuable comments.
2 The German slogan was "Mein Bauch gehört mir." Feminist activists and scholars have challenged this notion of the body as property; see Petchesky (1995).

treatments can no longer be endorsed by doctors; instead the decision about whether to undergo them is left to the patient.

Looking at prenatal genetic counseling, I argue that such professionally imposed self-determination does not empower patients but disables them. In genetic counseling, a pregnant woman is trained to become an informed and responsible consumer of prenatal tests. In order to accomplish this, the expert ascertains her risk status, adds a few more risks she had been unaware of, then lists her options—which basically boil down to whether or not to have a test such as an amniocentesis—and finally spells out the chances and risks associated with each option. The client discovers in the process that being pregnant means having to make decisions in the shadow of risk: either she risks delivering a disabled child, the counselor tells her, or she accepts the risk of an amniocentesis-induced miscarriage. And if the amniocentesis does not provide the green light she hopes for, she will have to consider terminating the pregnancy.

This new kind of self-determination does not increase the pregnant women's freedom. On the contrary, it entangles her in paralyzing contradictions. She is urged to make a decision that is mediated by technoscience and that requires professional services. Furthermore, to choose is compulsory, for even if the woman were to refuse to engage in decision making, it would be interpreted as a choice for the "no test" option and its precalculated risks. These characteristics of the new autonomy are at odds with precisely those abilities once implied by the notion of self-determination inasmuch as they tend to militate against freedom of action, trust in one's own senses, and independent judgment.

In this article I will first describe prenatal care as a service that burdens women with impossible decisions. I will then argue that decision making by doctors, geneticists, and other professional advisors is a new social technology and establish genetic counseling as a special site for its exploration. The main body of the argument will consist of a case-based analysis of the multiple paradoxes of taught self-determination. I intend to show that these paralyzing contradictions are the inevitable side effects of professional services whose product is "informed choice."

LOCATING TAUGHT DECISION MAKING IN PRENATAL CARE

In Western countries, the informed choice of the consumer has become a political and ethical sine qua non for prenatal diagnostics and genetic testing. As early as in the 1930s, businessman and eugenicist Frederick Osborne suggested that economic wealth and education would be more effective than coercive measures at establishing eugenics as a foundation for society. Genetic literacy, he hoped, would generate in parents a feeling of responsibility for the genetic makeup of their children (Weß 1989). In societies dominated by market economies, governing through freedom is obviously more effective than governing through direct control. Thus, in its meteoric transformation into a modern market society, even China—which was massively criticized for a eugenic draft law only ten years ago—now focuses its health policies on education and individual responsibility (Döring 2003).

In non-Western countries lacking a large, well-educated middle class, such as Mexico, India, and Peru, geneticists consider it their task to reduce the number of sick or disabled children and frankly tell their clients what to do (Wertz and Fletcher 2004). Autonomy, as it is celebrated in Western culture, is obviously granted to women only in those countries where the defining power of science and biomedicine over people's bodies and their very beings is predominant. Genetic literacy, or more generally, biomedical literacy, however, threatens knowledge based on experience and local cultures. Biomedicine has transformed the tender condition of expecting a child into an objectified biological state ascribed to women by experts. This diagnosed pregnancy is understood as a risk-laden reproductive process that must be monitored and managed according to professional guidelines.

Through the increasing use of techniques such as ultrasound and amniocentesis, this technologically mediated understanding of pregnancy has spread around the globe. When they seek medical care, women in nations like Vietnam and Nigeria are confronted with scientific objects such as the fetus, genes, and risks, as well as Western conceptions of health and responsibility. These ideas clash with local notions of what it means to have a child (Kaufert and O'Neil 1993; Duden, Schlumbohm, and Veit 2002; Inhorn 2002). For women who still rely on a phenomenologically grounded reality, the unborn is not an autonomous subject: it is a luminal being, beyond this space and time (Duden 2002b). Only birth reveals its reality (Duden 2002b; Gammeltoft 2007). For women not used to the Western hegemony of an instrumented reality, like the Vietnamese women interviewed by Tine Gammeltoft (2007) or the recent immigrants in Canada studied by Lisa Mitchell (2001), a sonogram provides neither the pleasures of seeing the baby nor the comfort of being reassured—as it does for European and North American women. In societies without the modern regime of insurance and prevention, the key concept of obstetrics, namely, statistically defined manageable risk, does not exist. Women in rural Mozambique, for example, consider envy the greatest threat to their pregnancies and therefore delay prenatal care in order to hide their state (Chapman 2003). For the Inuit women who are urged by physicians to give up births at home, "risk is the occasional threat of danger in childbirth accepted as part of a natural process" (Kaufert and O'Neil 1993, 50). But science and technology are power. Biomedical experts demand universal authority and suppress local knowledge and common sense (Davis-Floyd and Sargent 1997).[3] When the Inuit woman clarifies her point of view, "the physician dismisses her claims as irrelevant for a definition of risk which is objective, scientific, expressible in numbers" (Kaufert and O'Neil 1993, 50). Only those who submit to the rationality of fetal development and manageable risks are asked to make free choices—a freedom that stipulates distrust in one's own senses and a willed dependence on experts and machines. How paradoxical this kind of professionally and technologically mediated self-determination is will become clear in the course of my analysis.

PRENATAL CARE BURDENS WOMEN WITH IMPOSSIBLE DECISIONS

Modern prenatal care treats pregnant women not as expectant mothers but as managers of fetal risk profiles (Samerski 2007). Maternity books, midwives, obstetricians, and geneticists stress that becoming a responsible mother means having to make informed decisions. Pregnant women learn to heed dietary recommendations such as reducing coffee and avoiding raw

---

3 This suppression is never total; women always find ways to resist. See Abel and Browner 1998.

milk cheese; they are asked to select between delivery services—home birth or clinic? vaginal or caesarean? And, finally, in a decision with consequences, they have to choose which prenatal tests to undergo—regular ultrasound? a first-trimester test? amniocentesis?

It is particularly the decision about prenatal test options that gives women a headache (Friedrich, Henze, and Stemann-Acheampong 1998). Ever since the introduction of ultrasound scans and amniocentesis in the 1970s, a mother-to-be can no longer simply wait for her child to come. Either she must actively make an "informed decision" against testing or she will undergo prenatal checkups and enter into a state that sociologist Barbara Katz Rothman has called "tentative pregnancy" (Rothman 1987): if prenatal tests do not provide a green light, the expectant mother will have to consider an abortion.

In general, prenatal tests are offered to healthy women for a preventive checkup. The impetus of risk management turns anything that might happen to the woman and her coming child into a risk that she can either deliberately accept or guard against by testing. The simple fact that she is pregnant carries the risk that the child might have some congenital disorder (Samerski 2002). Furthermore, the expectant mother's age is fed into a statistical calculation to determine her risk of carrying a child with Down syndrome. A welter of other risks can follow. The German maternity passport, a handheld pregnancy record capturing all medical data, lists fifty-two factors that immediately classify a pregnant woman as being at risk. Among these are age of the woman over 35 or under 18, there being a genetic disease or disability among the woman's relatives, and the presence of a difficult family situation. The list is so broad and vague that roughly three out of four pregnancies are now diagnosed as being at risk (Schwarz and Schücking 2004, 25).

The attribution of risk transforms healthy women into patients who suffer a new iatrogenic anxiety: risk anxiety. Doctors cannot free patients from this fear. As a rule they refer to examinations as part of a process that will clarify and monitor the risk: ultrasound, maternal serum screening, and amniocentesis are by now widely practiced. However, doctors cannot truly recommend any of these options (Schmidtke 1995). For at least three reasons, risk management choices go beyond the traditional medical ground of diagnosis and therapy that so far has served as the basis for professional advice.

First of all, there is no cure. A positive test result can only provide reasons for terminating the pregnancy. Thus, any of the prenatal tests can lead the woman into a "one-way-street," as a genetic counselor aptly phrased it (quoted in Samerski 2002, 146), at the end of which the mother-to-be has to make an agonizing decision: either she deliberately carries an "abnormal" child to term or she terminates the pregnancy.

Second, tests cannot offer women the hoped-for reassurance that everything is all right. One can never determine whether the child is going to be healthy on the basis of a prenatal test. Of the various risks pregnant women are saddled with, most will still remain. Routine amniocentesis can only establish whether the chromosome set of the unborn is normal or not —which can bring unpleasant surprises, as a genetic counselor warns (quoted in Samerski 2002, 206).[4] Aberrations other than trisomy 21 might be detected, such as sex chromosome anomalies or changes with unforeseeable consequences.[5] A woman whose amniocentesis exhibited a chromosomal inversion learned that Down syndrome had been ruled out but that she now had an even higher risk that her child might be born with some other disability (Samerski 2002).[6]

Third, ruling out one risk often means having to accept another. Amniocentesis requires a puncture through the abdomen around the sixteenth week of pregnancy, which carries a 0.5–1 percent risk of inducing a miscarriage. Thus, only women classified as being at increased risk are eligible for testing. This selective criterion ensures, statistically, that the test does not cause harm at a higher rate than the rate at which it detects anomalies. Non-

---

4 In the event that there is a hereditary disease that runs in the family, a genetic test can also reveal whether the unborn has inherited the associated mutation or not. As is the case with cystic fibrosis, however, a positive genetic test result does not tell for certain if the child will be severely affected. There are children whose tests have revealed two severe mutations but who manifest only minor symptoms (Cystic Fibrosis Genotype-Phenotype Consortium 1993).

5 See the section titled "Self-Determination Mediated by Technoscience" in this article for more details on sex chromosome anomalies.

6 The test result showed an inversion in chromosome no. 5 with two breaking points. The counselor tried to calm the parents-to-be but had to inform them that, statistically, there was a 6 percent risk of a gene being affected that could lead to developmental disorders.

invasive screening procedures such as maternal serum screening and first-trimester screening aim at sifting those classified at increased risk out from the whole population of pregnant women. On the basis of the mother's hormone levels, her age, and, in the case of the first-trimester test, also the sonographically measured transparency of the fetal neck, the woman is statistically reclassified. She is placed in a new risk category, and the doctor then ascribes the frequency of worst-case scenarios for this statistical cohort to the woman as her personal risk. A pregnant woman aged 33 might get the test result that she runs a 1 : 275 chance of giving birth to a child with Down syndrome. Since physicians generally agree that 1 : 300 is a threshold for further testing, she will be offered an amniocentesis.[7]

Fourth, physicians are unable to recommend anything, as human geneticist Jörg Schmidtke (1995) has clearly pointed out, because they cannot establish a medical indication on the basis of calculated risks. Statistically, no pregnant woman is without risk, and every distinction between a low risk and a high risk is merely arbitrary. A risk attributed to a patient is not a diagnosis but a calculated probability that allows the expert to estimate the frequency with which something will happen in the artificial cohort in which the patient has been placed. Statistical figures do not say anything about specific cases but only estimate frequencies in populations. Consequently, because they cannot derive a professional "should" from statistical calculations, doctors hand decisions over to their patients.

FROM INFORMED CONSENT TO DECISION MAKING

In the 1970s, women activists and patients' rights activists fought hard to enforce the right to information. When the contraceptive pill was provided with a patient package insert, the first pharmaceutical product sold with this information, doctors were indignant over this intrusion into the doctor-patient relationship (Watkins 1998). In the 1980s, it became standard practice for German doctors to seek legal protection from potential future lawsuits by informing patients and obtaining their consent before an operation or

---

7   An alternative intervention, chorionic villus sampling, can be performed at an earlier stage of pregnancy. It yields the same results as amniocentesis but involves higher risks and is therefore not offered as routinely in Germany.

medical intervention (Beller 2000).[8] By signing a sheet, patients declare that they have been informed of the risks involved—for instance, of being blinded during an eye operation or of not waking up from the anesthetic after an appendectomy—and that they are willing to accept these risks.[9]

In prenatal care, however, the old rule of "doctor knows best" is superseded by "patient decides best." Doctors no longer prescribe a prenatal check or genetic test without making sure that the informed consent sheet is signed first. Instead, doctors confront their patients with a menu of options from which they—at their own risk—have to choose. Instead of prescribing the course of action they consider appropriate according to their professional standards, as had been the common practice for the "demigod in white" until the end of the twentieth century, doctors counsel their clients in order to guarantee their "informed choice." They enlighten women about their options, list their respective chances and risks, and, finally, appeal to the self-determination of the pregnant woman. In the formal and elaborate genetic counseling sessions that I observed for my study, women undergo a sixty- to ninety-minute crash course on chromosomes, genes, the probabilities of birth defects, their ominous portents about the newborn's future, and, finally, on a modern woman's obligation to bear the responsibility for her own decision making. "What I did want was for you to make a decision either for or against it," one counselor said to justify his hour-long explanation of the pros and cons of an amniocentesis.[10]

---

8 On the history of informed consent, see Faden and Beauchamp (1986) and Rothman (1991).

9 Adriana Petryna (2005) shows how the global industry of drug research uses the principle of informed consent, considered to protect human research subjects from coercion and abuse, for its own interest.

10 For my study on taught decision making in genetic counseling, I attended thirty genetic counseling sessions as a participant observer in three different counseling centers in Germany, all in accord with accepted human subject research protocols. Before the beginning of the session, clients were informed about my project and carefully asked for permission (in two cases they declined). During the sessions, I tape-recorded the conversations and made notes about gestures and facial expressions. The transcripts, from which I removed personal data, were made according to the GAT (Gesprächsanalytisches Transkriptionssystem) transcription rules for conversation analysis (Selting 1998). I analyzed the tran-

ANALYZING SELF-DETERMINATION IN PRENATAL CARE

Pregnant women's agonies as they make choices fraught with consequences on the basis of probabilistic data and predetermined options have been clearly described (Friedrich, Henze, and Stemann-Acheampong 1998; Rapp 1999). As empirical studies on risk perception and risk communication have shown, the designated decision makers struggle hard to make sense of numbers that, in principle, are senseless (Zuuren, van Schie, and van Baaren 1997; Kavanagh and Broom 1998; Rapp 1999). Thus, many women agonize over the decision they are expected to make. Rothman trenchantly describes the real consequences of an abstract rationale for a pregnant woman who "enters into a rational seeking of information and choices and finds herself trapped in a nightmare" (Rothman 1987, 181). In fact, a trio of German medical sociologists have called their empirical study on the decision pregnant women must make about undergoing amniocentesis "an impossible decision" (Friedrich, Henze, and Stemann-Acheampong 1998).

Nevertheless, the contradictions and dilemmas of genetic counseling have mostly been analyzed as a consequence of the clash between lay perceptions and expert information (Chapple, Campion, and May 1997; Rapp 1999; Browner et al. 2003) or of the incompatibility between clients' hope for certainty and the statistical nature of the conveyed information (Zuuren, van Schie, and van Baaren 1997) and between clients' search for advice and the principle of nondirectiveness (Williams, Alderson, and Farsides 2002). Thus, by identifying the social and cultural barriers preventing a "free choice" on the part of the client, most research on the subject has so far been guided by the assumption that, at least in principle, genetic counseling could enable informed decision making and thereby facilitate the exercise of autonomy.

Feminist scholars in particular have seen the new demand for decision making as a success in the struggle for emancipation. They honor choice and reproductive freedom as highly desirable values and welcome professional information and access to service options as prerequisites for the realization of these values (Rothenberg and Thomson 1994). Some feminist scholars, however, are troubled by the fact that it has become nearly impos-

---

scripts by following the qualitative approach of content analysis. For full detail, see Samerski (2002).

sible not to choose and have argued that choice can also be a new constraint (Rothman 1987; Gupta 2000). Sociologist William Arney has reversed the story of emancipation. He analyzed the shifting of responsibility from physicians to patients and the conceptualization of the patient as a decision maker not as a waning of professional power but as the result of increased biomedicalization. When definitions of health, influenced by systems theory, began to include psychological and social aspects, the medical profession extended its range of competence (Greco 1993). Redefined cybernetically, "life" became the new object of medicine, and its management the new goal. In order to make this all-embracing management possible, the patient was invited to be an active collaborator in the medical enterprise (Arney and Bergen 1984).

This argument has been reinforced by recent studies on governmentality. These studies see the call to exercise autonomy as a duty to manage oneself according to the rules of neoliberalism (Novas and Rose 2000; Rose 2001). Health is no longer seen as a something one enjoys or does not have but as something that is the result of responsible choices (Davison, Davey Smith, and Frankel 1991). Health "has come to represent, for the neo-liberal individual who has 'chosen' it, an 'objective' witness to his or her suitability to function as a free and rational agent" (Greco 1993, 369–70). However, what can be chosen in reality is not health itself but service options that promise to reduce health risks and enhance future well-being.

Education in risk awareness and the offer to manage these risks with professionally prescribed conduct creates "an obligation to act in the present in relation to the potential future that now comes into view" (Novas and Rose 2000, 486). This call to regard a possible future as a present threat that demands responsible decision making is particularly powerful when physicians attribute risks to their patients. In contrast to environmental or lifestyle risks, which are understood as hazards from the outside, embodied or corporeal risks indicate not only potential disasters in the future but also bodily "disorder in the present" (Kavanagh and Broom 1998, 442). After being classified as at risk, patients feel threatened and consider themselves on the verge of disease (Kavanagh and Broom 1998). Geneticization (Lippman 1991) aggravates the pathogenic effect of physicians' attributions. In the popular scientific imagination, genes crop up as causes for one's bodily features and personal peculiarities, be it a sibling's blue eyes and blond hair, a daughter's nail-biting habit, or an uncle's boozing (Duden and Samerski 2007).[11] Thus, when a geneticist diagnoses a gene for something or a genetic risk, one's fate appears to be sealed. Genes intimate a disaster that is already preprogrammed in one's own body (Samerski, forthcoming). Geneticization, therefore, transforms people into gene carriers who can be made responsible for managing their genetic risks and dispositions. It is this feeling of responsibility that urges woman to follow the rationale of riskmanagement: to opt for burdensomemonitoring, risky interventions, and preventing the gene from being passed on to their offspring (Hallowell 1999).

Focusing on "informed choices" in prenatal care, I argue that the call for responsible decision making under the shadow of genes and risks must be understood as a social engineering technique. It redefines self-determination so that it has to be facilitated by experts and mediated by technoscience. Whereas early feminists and their successors fought to liberate women from legal and political impositions, pregnant women today are highly dependent on experts and technology. My analysis of genetic counseling will illustrate how the professional imputation of this new autonomy makes women powerless while holding them responsible.

THE HISTORY OF PROFESSIONAL GUIDANCE AND GENETIC COUNSELING

Professional counseling, from investment advising at the Deutsche Bank to self-discovery courses in Tuscany, has become an integral part of contemporary society. Yet not even a century has passed since the first public counseling centers opened their doors in the United States and Europe. In Germany, the Weimar welfare state inaugurated the age of professional

---

11 Contemporary research on the complexity of the genome rebuts the hypothesis of genes as stable, functionally definable, and causal hereditary factors. Today many geneticists publicly admit what geneticist Wilhelm Johannsen, who coined the term "gene," clarified as early as 1913: the idea of material factors that determine characters and traits "must be dismissed not only as naïve, but also as totally misguided" (Johannsen 1913, 144; see also Beurton, Falk, and Rheinberger 2000). Despite this paradigm shift in genetics, "gene" remains a powerful term in colloquial language.

counseling.[12] After the new republic made it the task of the federal administration to guarantee the health and fitness of the population, clinics and counseling centers sprang up like mushrooms. Members of the working class especially were taught not to follow their habits, traditions, and common sense but to submit to science-based hygiene and health rules. Clean milk for the baby was not handed out to the young mother without instructions on hygiene and healthy food. Along with contraceptives, young couples were given lessons in sexology and eugenic family planning. Professional advice was one way to enforce upon citizens the behavioral adaptations demanded by an industrial society striving for progress (Sachße and Tennstedt 1988). In the past fifty years, professional counseling has advanced to become one of the most important social technologies. From infertility to parenthood, from studying to drug habits, from sickness to death and bereavement—today, every conceivable situation in life presents a potential need for counseling. In contrast to expert guidance in the 1920s, contemporary counseling no longer aims to adapt the behavior of citizens to the societal plans of economic, medical, and sociopolitical experts. Rather, as my analysis of genetic counseling will show, the self-determination lessons of today set up the framework within which citizens are supposed to understand themselves and make their own decisions. The goal is no longer standardized behavior but much more subtle, risk-guided, and option-oriented voluntary decision making.

An especially telling example of such an attempt to palm off the choice between preprogrammed options and precalculated risks as an act of self-determination is that of genetic counseling. A consultation with a new kind of educator who specializes in interpreting chromosome charts and biostatistics and who has mastered communication techniques is supposed to assist a pregnant woman in making a so-called autonomous decision about prenatal testing options—and perhaps, subsequently, also about the option to terminate her pregnancy. The explicit goal of this one-to-two-hour crash course in biostatistics and genetics is not to comply with professionally prescribed conduct but to offer professional assistance to individuals making decisions (Berufsverband Medizinische Genetik e.V. 1996; see also Ad Hoc Committee on Genetic Counseling 1975).

---

12 On the history of counseling as a public service, see Samerski (2002).

In the early 1970s, when genetic counseling was reestablished in Germany, it was still seen as a eugenic measure. The explicit goal of the geneticist's advice was to prevent the birth of a handicapped child (Wendt 1975). Before the introduction of amniocentesis in the early 1970s, genetic counselors could do nothing more than apply Gregor Mendel's rules to the hypothetical pairing of their clients in order to discourage the "unfit" from having children. Most people had no use for such genetic prognostication, and demand for such consultations was low. Until the late 1970s, physicians still complained about the fact that healthy people did not visit the doctor. Not only genetic counseling but also preventive measures such as prenatal care and cancer prevention initially met with limited interest (Theile 1977, viii).

Today, in contrast, physicians no longer complain about the general population's lack of knowledge regarding health matters but rather about the insufficient number of counseling centers. Information about the various handicaps and diseases a newborn might have has since become an everyday part of prenatal care.[13] Genetic counseling has been transformed from making hereditary prognostications into a service industry selling information, knowledge, and reassurance as the essential raw materials for informed decision making about prenatal test options. The goal of such counseling sessions is no longer the eugenic prevention of abnormal people but the creation of products that satisfy individual preferences (Ad Hoc Committee on Genetic Counseling 1975; Berufsverband Medizinische Genetik e.V. 1996).

---

13 The German Kassenärztliche Bundesvereinigung counts roughly fifty thousand genetic counseling sessions—which also include nonprenatal genetic counseling—every year, and seventy to eighty thousand fetal karyotyping tests (Schmidtke, Pabst, and Nippert 2005). This means that quite a number of women undergo an amniocentesis without regular genetic counseling. Counseling for routine prenatal diagnostics is usually left to obstetricians.

TAUGHT SELF-DETERMINATION IN GENETIC COUNSELING

The following is a qualitative analysis of taught self-determination in genetic counseling sessions. This analysis is based on thirty observed and recorded genetic counseling sessions in three different counseling centers in Germany in 1997, all in accordance with accepted human subject research protocols (for the full details, see Samerski 2002). All quotations below are translated from these German-language transcripts.

Whether in Berlin or San Francisco, the goal and principles of genetic counseling are the same; even the structure of the sessions and some of the formulations are comparable (Rapp 1999; Wertz and Fletcher 2004). What differs is the counselor's educational background. In the United States and Canada, a master's degree program has turned genetic counseling into a growing profession almost completely dominated by women. By contrast, German genetic counselors are men and women with MDs and five years of advanced training in molecular biology, genetic epidemiology, chromosome preparation, and counseling techniques.[14]

In Germany, it was only in the 1990s that the goal of autonomous decision making and the principle of nondirectiveness gained full acceptance (Waldschmidt 1996). Professional guidelines for the field were formulated in 1996 and are still valid today (Berufsverband Medizinische Genetik e.V. 1996). Therefore, neither the theory nor the practice of prenatal genetic counseling has significantly changed within the past ten years.[15]

SELF-DETERMINATION AS SERVICE DEPENDENCY

The autonomous decision making that genetic counseling aims at does not presuppose any freedom of action on the part of the woman. Her only activity consists in deciding what she wants to consume. Today a positive

---

14 Among the five genetic counselors I observed, only one was a woman. This ratio is not representative.

15 For a brief and recent overview of the goals, definitions, and practical aspects of genetic counseling in Germany, see Zerres (2003).

pregnancy test confirms, above all, a woman's need for services and products. After receiving positive results from a pregnancy test or if they have missed a period, women are expected to see a doctor. There, with medical authorization, they officially become clients with special needs—needs that were alien to women one or two generations ago. Countless magazines, courses, and books offer advice on pre- and post- natal bonding, a holistic pregnancy experience, and the most experientially rich ways of giving birth. Consuming vitamin products, abstaining from coffee, and completing stress-management courses are some of the many techniques that doctors recommend for the management of fetal development. The transformation of the pregnant woman into a uterine system clearly makes her into a needy consumer of products and services (Duden 1993; Taylor 2000).

But even if the pregnant woman does selflessly transform herself into a uterine system, she cannot simply wait for her child to arrive. It is increasingly unlikely that her obstetrician still belongs to the maligned old guard and will whisk her without much ado through the various prenatal tests. Instead, with much personalized attention, she will be told of the risks of bearing children and the possibilities of prenatal quality control. Yet, with regard to the pregnant women's hope—namely, a healthy child—there is no consumer option. Prenatal test results merely refine calculations of risk or exclude specific diagnoses within an unlimited sea of possibilities of frightening outcomes. And, in the case of a positive test result, the only "therapy" is terminating the pregnancy.

There is a gulf between the offerings of the service industry and a woman's longing. Thus, genetic counselors have to translate the hopes and fears of pregnant women into questions that are compatible with their scientific expertise. Hence, the vague fear that the child might be "not normal" (Press et al. 1998) is turned into the specific quest for excluding, say, the possibility of Down syndrome. And the growing sense of motherly care for her future child is perverted into a woman's sense of responsibility for risk management.

The woman quoted below still grieves about having had a late abortion after an ultrasound test detected anencephalus. Now she wants to make sure that she is doing everything she can to prevent this from happening again:

Woman: Yes, so he [the obstetrician] recommended that we come here for counseling, and . . . that this might reassure us a bit, or . . . yes.

Counselor: Yes, mhm.
Woman: Well, for me it's more a matter of doing what I can.

In the very next sentence, however, the counselor reworks the woman's hope for precautionary measures into a need for information about statistical probabilities. He interprets her desire to "do what she can" as a request to find out the recurrence rate of the problem.

Counselor: Mhm, yes. So, pertaining to the question, if I may help: recurrence, no recurrence.

The counselor informs his anxious client about various pregnancy-related risks. He covers the so-called base risk in general, her age-specific risk of carrying a child with Down syndrome, and the risk of neural tube defects in particular. Anencephalus belongs to the latter, as he explains, which is categorized as multifactorial. He lists several other diseases that belong to this category, along with their occurrence risks.

Counselor: The probability of recurrence is statistically . . . 4 to 6 percent. Or after a child with congenital heart defect, 2 percent. And after a child with a neural tube defect, roughly 4 percent.
Women: Mhm.
Counselor: Statistical probability of recurrence.

During the session the woman mentions an early miscarriage she had fifteen years ago. Consequently, the counselor enlightens the woman about the possibility of chromosomal rearrangements linked to an increased risk for miscarriages. As the counselor frankly admits, there is no single reason to suspect that the couple should have such a chromosomal rearrangement. Nevertheless, he offers a blood test to exclude this possibility in order to give the couple some reassurance. The woman, willing to submit to whatever is possible, gratefully accepts the expert's offer.

 The statistical probabilities that the counselor lists do not add an iota to his client's knowledge about the health of her future child. But, even worse, the counselor opens up a new range of possible disasters and then offers a test to exclude one of those fearsome possibilities. In order to do what she can, the woman opts for the test. Counseling teaches women not to hope for what they want but to want only that for which a prefabricated option exists.

SELF-DETERMINATION MEDIATED BY TECHNOSCIENCE

Until a generation or two ago, pregnant women had nothing to decide about their children-to-be. They were careful not to harm their unborn by bad thoughts or sights, but the outcome of the pregnancy remained always uncertain (Duden 2002b). However, the emergence of a developmental-biological way of thinking and the techniques to visually represent the unborn child have transformed pregnancy into a developmental-biological process. Once the ideal value, namely, the normal course of pregnancy, could be predetermined, it seemed necessary to subject the contents of the female body to technical surveillance. The focus of medical attention shifted from the pregnant woman to the uterine system in the service of biological development, whose norm-oriented progress was to be read from computer screens and laboratory findings. And, if the experts determined with ultrasound scanners and microscopes that the measured actual value deviated from the calculated ideal value, the further development of the fetus was called into question (Oakley 1984; Duden 1993).

When pregnancy no longer refers to the expectation of a child but rather to an optimized reproductive process, a woman can no longer trust her senses. The technological reconstruction of reality demands that she doubt her own corporeality. Barbara Duden (1993) has described how the sonographic depiction of the fetus tempts one to mistake the visual representation of the child for the unborn child itself. The rituals of prenatal care teach the woman to ascribe to herself developmental stages and hormone levels—technological abstractions that she is supposed to consider more real than what she feels and can see with her own eyes and experience physically.

The counselor's lessons challenge the client to take a further step in this disembodiment. The woman is encouraged to believe not only that the shadow on the computer screen shows what is going on with her today but also that genetic models and probability calculations can predict what might happen tomorrow. Risk curves, electrophoretic gels, and chromosome charts claim to provide evidence not only about the veiled fruit of her womb but also about her own veiled future.

When the counselor shows a client the results of an amniocentesis, he places a piece of paper on the table, on which small, wormlike objects, arranged according to size, can be seen: a so-called karyotype—chromosomes that, at a very specific stage of cell development, are processed, stained, photographed under a microscope, and subsequently sorted. In these little worms the pregnant woman is supposed to glimpse the fate of her coming child. The geneticist explains to her that the hereditary material, the genes, is packed into the chromosomes.

Counselor: So, the chromosomes are important [smiles]. . . . They influence us all of our lives. And we have them in all of our cells. . . . So, the genes are strung along these chromosomes like beads on a necklace, a thousand or more on a large chromosome.

In the lower right section of the illustration, a red squiggle calls attention to a trio of chromosomes, three small clumps, whereas all the others are stuck together in pairs: Trisomy 21, the chromosomal evidence for Down syndrome. Should the client's amniocentesis yield a karyotype like this one, she could opt to interrupt her pregnancy, the counselor offers.

It was only fifty years ago that scientists were heatedly arguing about the number of human chromosomes; by now, a page covered with forty-six, or sometimes forty-five or forty-seven, wormlike objects is so impressive that it easily imposes itself between the expectant mother and her unborn child. Today, the fears of pregnant women crystalize around the third chromosome 21, the laboratory result for Down syndrome: it evokes her anxiety that the child might not be "normal" and thus not be socially accepted, and it fuels her greatest fears of having to provide life-long care (Press et al. 1998). These worries of pregnant women are legitimate. What is dangerous, however, is that today these fears are bound up with technological abstractions; the biochemical laboratory results and calculations of risk can seem to be of such significance for the future that an expectant mother regards the fate of her child as sealed even before it has been born.

It is estimated that over 90 percent of women terminate their pregnancies if a finding of trisomy 21 is made. Interviews show that, for many women, the prediction of mental retardation is a reason for abortion because they fear social hostility (Press et al. 1998). On the basis of the lab result, however, no one can predict to what extent the child will actually be impaired. The intellectual capacities of children with Down syndrome vary greatly, with the range of IQ adjoining those considered normal (Canning and Pueschel 1995, 80). As geneticists have reported to me, many women also opt for an abortion in the event of sex chromosome anomalies, for instance, in the event of Turner syndrome or Klinefelter syndrome. Yet there are men and women who learn that they have such a syndrome only because of incomplete development at puberty or even much later when they discover that they cannot have children. In the case of Klinefelter, it is even assumed that roughly 90 percent of an estimated forty to eighty thousand cases in Germany have not yet been discovered (Deutsche Klinefelter-Syndrom Vereinigung e.V. 2005, 10).

STATISTICAL FORTUNE TELLING

During the counseling session, women are well informed about possibilities, probabilities, and potentialities. Genetic counselors' expertise enables them to speculate about what might happen and to put this "might" into a statistical frame. Almost everything genetic counselors tell clients about their pregnancies and their expected children is based on statistical calculations (Rapp 1999; Samerski 2002). It is common to speak of "your risk" and "individual risk" and to equate this figure explicitly or implicitly with personal insecurity.

Counselor: If security is important to you, you have no other choice but amniocentesis.
Woman: Yes.
Counselor: Because the triple-test, as I said, only yields an individual risk, but no security.

Through such colloquial formulations, genetic counselors suggest that risk figures can gauge the prospect of a healthy baby. This fuels a fundamental misunderstanding: the misleading presumption that a doctor-attested risk estimates the degree of threat to a patient. Risk figures can predict nothing about an individual woman, however. The geneticist has not diagnosed any health threat or physical ailment but has merely placed the client in a statistical category based on one characteristic, namely, her age or a test result. He then ascribes the probabilistic characteristics of this fictional cohort of women in terms of an individual woman's risk.

Human genetics has altered the understanding of illness and the meaning of diagnosis. Previously, it was not possible to make a diagnosis without a patient. Today, however, a genetic finding is considered a diagnosis regardless of whether anything is wrong with the patient—or even if that patient has not yet been born. On the grounds of a biochemical or chromosomal anomaly, geneticists place the unborn child in a diagnostic category. They present the average development of this group to a client as the future prognosis for her child. However, as average values and probabilities cannot be valid for an individual, geneticists make no concrete statements about either the woman sitting in front of them or the unborn baby. Being urged to see rhyme and reason in abstract numbers, clients interpret them in very diverse, often bizarre ways. Some, irrespective of the number, feel certain that it will hit them, whereas others expect to be lucky (Parsons and Atkinson 1992). One woman, being warned about her high risk for having a child with muscular dystrophy, which was framed in terms of one out of ten, was relieved. "What good is that to me, I would never want a load of children anyway, my mother had six" (quoted in Parsons and Atkinson 1992, 443).

Most women, however, are bewildered by the various risks pinned on them (see Kavanagh and Broom 1998; Samerski 2002). Expecting their doctor to say something concrete and tangible about them, they inevitably understand genetic risk as a diagnosis, a personal threat that then hangs over their present-day lives like a Damoclean sword. No matter which examination the woman chooses, none will ever be able to restore the peace of mind she might have had before undergoing the series of tests. The medical attribution of risks to healthy people has therefore become a major pathogen. Predicting future disaster transforms the body into a time bomb (Lock 1998), and statistical calculations have turned the pregnant woman's state of happy expectation into one of foreboding (Rothman 1987; Samerski 2002).

Modern fortune tellers are thus no longer astrologers but bureaucrats. They no longer interpret the positions of the heavenly bodies but make their predictions on the basis of statistical tables and calculations of probability.

Furthermore, in contrast to astrologers, who understand their patrons as people born under a certain star, geneticists do not; they cannot treat their clients as persons. Their expertise is based on the statistical homogenization of individuals and the probabilistic characteristics of fictive cohorts. The fact that they address the client personally in colloquial language merely obscures the gulf between the woman before them and the data record from which their statements derive. Yet, not only do they transform the woman into a risk profile, they also demand of her that she do the same to her unborn child. She, as well, is supposed to understand the being that will become her kin as a risk profile, as a faceless member of various risk categories.

COMPULSORY SELF-DETERMINATION

Technical procedures that open up new examination and treatment possibilities also radically alter what has previously existed and been regarded as self-evident. The freedom to leave to fate that which one can neither determine nor decide has been undermined by such technologies as genetic testing, artificial insemination, and ultrasound scanning. The knowledge of the unforeseeability of what tomorrow will bring yields to the illusion of control. Once prenatal tests became a generally accessible service option, they make the decision about whether to take advantage of them practically unavoidable. Doctors who cannot prove that they have comprehensively informed their pregnant patients about the risks of childbearing and the range of services offered by prenatal medicine have been sentenced by courts to pay child support in cases where the newborn child did not meet the standards of normality. Thus, the justice system has imposed upon physicians a duty to counsel their patients.[16] For women, it has become increasingly difficult to maintain an attitude in which being pregnant is synonymous with expectation. As Duden (2002a) has clearly shown, historically pregnancy has not described a biological condition but rather a particular attitude on the part of the woman: a somatic stance, experienced by the sense of touch and oriented toward the birth of a child. She concludes that historically there has been no objectifiable state of pregnancy "but rather women who

---

16 On the legal system in relation to prenatal medicine in Germany, see Pap (1995).

felt pregnant" (Duden 2002a, 64). The now-antiquated German expression *guter Hoffnung sein* (being of good hope) emphasizes this particular attitude on the part of the pregnant woman, or her attitude toward the child she is expecting.

As one client in a genetic counseling session put it, a test that in the vast majority of cases can only serve to provide grounds for terminating the pregnancy is "out of the question" for a woman who is expecting. A woman in her mid-thirties is referred by her obstetrician to a geneticist because her sister has a severe handicap. As this particular disability cannot be diagnosed prenatally, the matter is quickly closed.

However, in the course of performing his educational duties, the counselor informs the pregnant woman of her age risk and suggests the possibility of amniocentesis. The woman is confused because she has not considered such a test.

Woman: But all the same, I haven't even thought about whether I would even consider it.
Counselor: Well, it . . . doesn't necessarily have to be decided upon today
Woman: No, for me, I have to say, that's not a matter for discussion.

This response, however, is apparently not an option in this age of self-determination. The counselor insists that she must make an informed decision.

Counselor: I'm not really sure—I might have brought you into a conflict. Of course, that was not my intention. What I did want was for you to make a decision either for or against it.

The counselor cannot reconcile his attitude with that of the woman, for whom such a test is simply out of the question and who therefore rejects weighing the risks and benefits involved. She is expecting and trusts in God, as she says. For her, there is nothing to decide. In representing amniocentesis as an option worth considering and about which she should decide, the counselor has destroyed her stance. Expecting a child is not an option to be weighed.

Genetic counselors cannot be accused of pressuring clients to undergo tests. On the contrary, they offer pregnant women the possibility of taking advantage of these procedures but also the option of abstaining from them. Yet it was precisely this manner of presenting what was beyond consideration as an option that confused this particular woman. During the counseling session, the possibility of undergoing amniocentesis and perhaps of aborting the fetus stand as equally weighted alternatives, which until now had not required any decision by the pregnant woman: she was bringing her child into the world, with no ifs, ands, or buts. In the same way in which he calculates the risks a test may involve, the counselor also calculates in advance the risks to which the woman exposes herself should she choose not to undergo amniocentesis. The counselor has modeled her future in such a way that any possible outcome could be seen as a consequence of her decision.

There is a whole series of studies analyzing the so-called reproductive decision in terms of decision theory (Frets et al. 1990)—that is, according to a model that is supposed to make management decisions calculable. This statistical model of decision making is now propagated as a set of instructions on how decisions in general ought to be made (Hammond, Keeney, and Raiffa 1999). Professional decision-making aids such as genetic counseling are shaped by this new understanding of decisions (Samerski 2002). The visual representation of the decision-making model described here is the decision tree: there are at least two options to choose from, and both have many possible and variously probable outcomes.

This model presents the pregnant woman with a trap: the decision trap. Be it a miscarriage as a result of the amniocentesis or a child with Down Syndrome—all at once she is responsible, even for things that she cannot influence. Simply being pregnant, as uncomplicatedly as one could still be a generation or two ago, is no longer possible. The decision trap turns the state of expectation into a self-determined decision to accept the risks involved in giving birth to a handicapped child. Another counselor explicitly tells his client that today a woman has only herself to blame if she simply gives in to fate. While he does not compel her to take the test, he makes it clear that she should know what she is doing if she chooses not to do so. After informing her of her age risk of giving birth to a child with Down syndrome, he states frankly:

Counselor: In any event you know, and if you don't want to simply bow down to fate, you don't have to.

Thus, it is not only genetic manipulation that turns a child into a planned product. The manufactured person—commonly presented as a horror scenario for the future—is already becoming a reality through the decision trap. Soon every child will owe its existence to a self-determined decision on the part of its mother—and this does not refer to her wish to have a child or her decision to continue with an unwanted pregnancy but to her weighing of risks, her managerial decision making.

GENETIC COUNSELING AS A TECHNIQUE OF SOCIAL ENGINEERING

In the twentieth century, knowledge and competencies, in order to be valuable, had to be acquired under the technical supervision of experts and evaluated by their scientific standards (Illich 1987). In the twenty-first century, not only knowledge and skills but also deliberation and decision making are being refashioned as scientific objects. Freedom, choice, and autonomy are being redefined in a way that requires scientific input and guidance services in order for them to be appropriately exercised. Counseling for autonomous decision making should therefore be analyzed as an encroachment of professional power on deliberation and decision.

In contrast to the "tyranny of the experts" (Lieberman 1970), when paternalistic professionals expected compliance from their clients, the goal of teaching decision making is not obedience but the production of "responsible citizens" who will voluntarily submit to the logic of risk and risk management. In this light, genetic counseling can be understood as a technique of social engineering. The decisions pregnant women are being asked to make are very similar to an investment decision when speculating on the stock market: they are supposed to choose among various preselected options and to be prepared to accept the associated calculated risks. They are asked to anticipate their coming child in terms of a distribution of possible outcomes and to follow the rationale of decision theory for reducing risks and making the optimal choice. Thus, this study on professionally taught self-determination ties into social science studies that analyze the emergence of a new managerial subjectivity in an epoch of risk calculation and biopolitics (Greco 1993; Novas and Rose 2000; Rose 2001). It reveals in detail what it means when "life itself," as Nikolas Rose puts it, enters the domain of politics and choice (Rose 2001). As genetic counseling exemplifies, prenatal decision making does not increase a woman's autonomy, nor does it bring her closer to her desire: a healthy or at least "normal" child. Instead, "the pregnant woman is both disempowered and held responsible at the same time" (Balsamo 1996, 110). She learns that trusting her own senses is deceptive and that she is considered responsible only if she submits to laboratory results, risk calculations, and managerial decision making. This is the social function of taught decision making: it makes clients powerless and responsible—even for things beyond their control.

REFERENCES

Abel, Emily K., and Carole H. Browner. 1998. "Selective Compliance with Biomedical Authority and the Uses of Experiential Knowledge." In Pragmatic Women and Body Politics, ed. Margaret Lock and Patricia A. Kaufert, 310–26. Cambridge: Cambridge University Press.

Ad Hoc Committee on Genetic Counseling. 1975. "Genetic Counseling." In American Journal of Human Genetics 27(2):240–42.

Arney, William Ray, and Bernard J. Bergen. 1984. Medicine and the Management of Living: Taming the Last Great Beast. Chicago: University of Chicago Press.

Balsamo, Anne. 1996. Technologies of the Gendered Body: Reading Cyborg Women. Durham, NC: Duke University Press.

Beller, Fritz K. 2000. "Informed Consent: Patientenaufklärung oder Patientenberatung?" [Informed consent: Patient information or patient counseling?] In Speculum 18(1):6–11.

Berufsverband Medizinische Genetik e.V. [Professional Association of Medical Genetics]. 1996. "Leitlinien zur Erbringung Humangenetischer Leistungen: 1, Leitlinien zur Genetischen Beratung" [Guidelines for carrying out human genetic services: 1, Guidelines for genetic counseling]. In Medizinische Genetik [Medical genetics] 8(3):1–2.

Beurton, Peter J., Raphael Falk, and Hans-Jörg Rheinberger. 2000. The Concept of the Gene in Development and Evolution: Historical and Epistemological Perspectives. Cambridge: Cambridge University Press.

Browner, Carole H., Mabel H. Preloran, Maria Christina Casado, Harold N. Bass, and Ann P.Walker. 2003. "Genetic Counseling Gone Awry: Miscommunication between Prenatal Genetic Service Providers and Mexican-Origin Clients." In Social Science and Medicine 56(9):1933–46.

Canning, Claire D., and Siegfried M. Pueschel. 1995. "Zum Verlauf der Entwicklung des Kindes: Ein Überblick" [On the course of child development: An overview]. In *Down*-Syndrom: Für Eine Bessere Zukunft [Down Syndrome: For a better future], ed. Siegfried M. Pueschel, 78–83. Stuttgart: TRIAS.

Chapman, Rachel R. 2003. "Endangering Safe Motherhood in Mozambique: Prenatal Care as Pregnancy Risk." In Social Science and Medicine 57(2):355–74.

Chapple, Alison, Peter Campion, and Carl May. 1997. "Clinical Terminology: Anxiety and Confusion amongst Families Undergoing Genetic Counseling." In Patient Education and Counseling 32(1–2):81–91.

Cystic Fibrosis Genotype-Phenotype Consortium. 1993. "Correlation between Genotype and Phenotype in Patients with Cystic Fibrosis." In New England Journal of Medicine 329(18):1308–13.

Davis-Floyd, Robbie E., and Carolyn F. Sargent, eds. 1997. Childbirth and Authoritative Knowledge: Cross-Cultural Perspectives. Berkeley: University of California Press.

Davison, Charlie, George Davey Smith, and Stephen Frankel. 1991. "Lay Epidemiology and the Prevention Paradox: The Implications of Coronary Candidacy for Health Education." In Sociology of Health and Illness 13(1):1–19.

Deutsche Klinefelter-Syndrom Vereinigung e.V. [German Klinefelter Syndrome Association e.V.]. 2005. "Klinefelter-Syndrom: Fragen und Antworten" [Klinefelter syndrome: Questions and answers]. 4th completely revised ed. Brochure. German Klinefelter Syndrome Association e.V., Falkenstein.

Döring, Ole. 2003. "Yousheng, Eugenik in China: Wo ist das ethische Problem?" [Yousheng, eugenics in China: What is the ethical problem?]. In Veranstaltungsdokumentation: "GuteGene—schlechteGene" [Documentary report:"Good genes—bad genes"]. Bundeszentrale für politische Bildung [Federal Office for Political Education]. Bremen. September. http://www.bpb.de/veranstaltungen/0WT01Q .html.

Duden, Barbara. 1993. Disembodying Women: Perspectives on Pregnancy and the Unborn. Trans. Lee Hoinacki. Cambridge, MA: Harvard University Press.

— 2002a. Die Gene im Kopf—Der Fötus im Bauch [Genes in the mind—fetus in the belly]. Hanover: Offizin.
— 2002b. "Zwischen 'Wahrem Wissen' und Prophetie: Konzeptionen des Ungeborenen" [Between "true knowledge" and prophecy: Conceptions of the unborn]. In Duden, Schlumbohm, and Veit 2002, 11–48.
Duden, Barbara, and Silja Samerski. 2007. "'Pop-Genes': An Investigation of 'the Gene' in Popular Parlance." In Biomedicine as Culture: Instrumental Practices, Technoscientific Knowledge, and New Modes of Life, ed. Regula V. Burri and Joseph Dumit, 167–89. New York: Routledge.
Duden, Barbara, Jürgen Schlumbohm, and Patrice Veit, eds. 2002. Geschichte des Ungeborenen: Zur Erfahrungs- und Wissenschaftsgeschichte der Schwangerschaft, 17.–20. Jahrhundert [The history of the unborn: About the history of experience and the history of science of pregnancy, seventeenth to twentieth century]. Göttingen: Vandenhoeck & Ruprecht.
Faden, Ruth R., and Tom L. Beauchamp. 1986. A History and Theory of Informed Consent. New York: Oxford University Press.
Frets, Petra G., Hugo J. Duivenvoorden, Frans Verhage, Martinus F. Niermeijer, Sophie M. M. van de Berge, and Hans Galjaard. 1990. "Factors Influencing the Reproductive Decision after Genetic Counseling." In American Journal of Medical Genetics 35(4):496–502.
Friedrich, Hannes, Karl H. Henze, and Susanne Stemann-Acheampong. 1998. Eine unmögliche Entscheidung: Pränataldiagnostik; Ihre Psychosozialen Voraussetzungen und Folgen [An impossible decision: Prenatal diagnostics; its psycho-social preconditions and consequences]. Berlin: VWB.
Gammeltoft, Tine. 2007. "Sonography and Sociality: Obstetrical Ultrasound Imaging in Urban Vietnam." In Medical Anthropology Quarterly 21(2):133–53.
Greco, Monica. 1993. "Psychosomatic Subjects and the 'Duty to BeWell': Personal Agency within Medical Rationality." In Economy and Society 22(3):357–72.
Grossmann, Atina. 1995. Reforming Sex: The German Movement for Birth Control and Abortion Reform, 1920–1950. New York: Oxford University Press.

Gupta, Jyotsna Agnihotri. 2000. New Reproductive Technologies, Women's Health and Autonomy: Freedom or Dependency? New Delhi: Sage.

Hallowell, Nina. 1999. "Doing the Right Thing: Genetic Risk and Responsibility." In Sociology of Health and Illness 21(5):597–621.

Hammond, John S., Ralph L. Keeney, and Howard Raiffa. 1999. Smart Choices: A Practical Guide to Making Better Decisions. Boston: Harvard Business School Press.

Illich, Ivan. 1987. "Disabling Professions." In Disabling Professions, ed. Ivan Illich, Irving K. Zola, John McKnight, Jonathan Caplan, and Harley Shaiken, 11–39. New York: Marion Boyars.

Inhorn, Marcia C. 2002. "The 'Local' Confronts the 'Global': Infertile Bodies and New Reproductive Technologies in Egypt." In Infertility around the Globe: New Thinking on Childnessness, Gender, and Reproductive Technologies, ed. Marcia C. Inhorn and Frank van Balen, 263–82. Berkeley: University of California Press.

Johannsen, Wilhelm. 1913. Elemente der Exakten Erblichkeitslehre [Elements of the exact theory of heritability]. 2nd rev. and extended ed. Jena: Fischer.

Kaufert, Patricia A., and John O'Neil. 1993. "Analysis of a Dialogue on Risks in Childbirth: Clinicians, Epidemiologists, and Inuit Women." In Knowledge, Power and Practice: The Anthropology of Medicine and Everyday Life, ed. Shirley Lindenbaum and Margaret Lock, 32–54. Berkeley: University of California Press.

Kavanagh, Anne M., and Dorothy H. Broom. 1998. "Embodied Risk: My Body, Myself?" In Social Science and Medicine 46(3):437–44.

Lieberman, Jethro K. 1970. The Tyranny of the Experts: How Professionals Are Closing the Open Society. New York: Walker.

Lippman, Abby. 1991. "Prenatal Genetic Testing and Screening: Constructing Needs and Reinforcing Inequities." American Journal of Law and Medicine 17(1–2):15–50.

Lock, Margaret. 1998. "Breast Cancer: Reading the Omens." In Anthropology Today 14(4):7–16.

Lupton, Deborah. 1995. The Imperative of Health: Public Health and the Regulated Body. London: Sage.

Mitchell, Lisa M. 2001. Baby's First Picture: Ultrasound and the Politics of Fetal Subjects. Toronto: University of Toronto Press.

Novas, Carlos, and Nikolas Rose. 2000. "Genetic Risk and the Birth of the Somatic Individual." In Economy and Society 29(4):485–513.
Oakley, Ann. 1984. The Captured Womb: A History of the Medical Care of Pregnant Women. Oxford: Basil Blackwell.
Pap, Michael. 1995. "Genetische Beratung und Nichtdirektivität im Licht der zivilrechtlichen Haftungsrechtsprechung" [Genetic counseling and nondirectiveness in the light of civil law liability jurisdiction]. In Zwischen Neutralität und Weisung: Zur Theorie und Praxis von Beratung in der Humangenetik [Between neutrality and instructions: On the theory and practice of counseling in human genetics], ed. Erhard Ratz, 51–56. München: Evangelischer Presseverband für Bayern. Parsons, Evelyn, and Paul Atkinson. 1992. "Lay Constructions of Genetic Risk." In Sociology of Health and Illness 14(4):437–55.
Petchesky, Rosalind Pollack. 1995. "The Body as Property: A Feminist Revision." In Conceiving the New World Order: The Global Politics of Reproduction, ed. Faye D. Ginsburg and Rayna Rapp, 387–406. Berkeley: University of California Press.
Petryna, Adriana. 2005. "Ethical Variability: Drug Development and Globalizing Clinical Trials." In American Ethnologist 32(2):183–97.
Press, Nancy A., Carole H. Browner, Diem Tran, Christine Morton, and Barbara LeMaster. 1998. "Provisional Normalcy and 'Perfect Babies': Pregnant Women's Attitudes toward Disability in the Context of Prenatal Testing." In Reproducing Reproduction: Kinship, Power, and Technological Innovation, ed. Sarah Franklin and Helena Ragoné, 46–65. Philadelphia: University of Pennsylvania Press.
Rapp, Rayna. 1999. Testing Women, Testing the Fetus: The Social Impact of Amniocentesis in America. New York: Routledge.
Rose, Nikolas. 2001. "The Politics of Life Itself." In Theory, Culture and Society 18(6):1–30.
Rothenberg, Karen H., and Elizabeth J. Thomson, eds. 1994. Women and Prenatal Testing: Facing the Challenges of Genetic Technology. Columbus: Ohio State University Press.
Rothman, Barbara K. 1987. The Tentative Pregnancy: Prenatal Diagnosis and the Future of Motherhood. New York: Penguin.
Rothman, David J. 1991. Strangers at the Bedside: A History of How Law and Bioethics Transformed Medical Decision Making. New York: Basic.

Sachße, Christoph, and Florian Tennstedt. 1988. Geschichte der Armenfürsorge in Deutschland [The history of poor relief in Germany]. Vol. 2, In Fürsorge und Wohlfahrtspflege, 1871–1929 [Relief and welfare work, 1871–1929]. Stuttgart: Kohlhammer.

Samerski, Silja. 2002. Die Verrechnete Hoffnung: Von der selbstbestimmten Entscheidung durch genetische Beratung [The mathematization of hope: On autonomous decision making through genetic counseling]. Münster: Westfälisches Dampfboot.

— 2007. "The 'Decision Trap':How Genetic Counseling Transforms Pregnant Women into Managers of Foetal Risk Profiles." In Gendered Risks, ed. Pat O'Malley and Kelly Hannah-Moffat, 55–74. London: Routledge Cavendish.

— Forthcoming. "The Symbolic Fallout of Gene Talk." In Disclosure Dilemmas: Ethical Issues of Information in Genetic Counselling, ed. Christoph Rehmann-Sutter and Hansjakob Müller. London: Ashgate.

Schmidtke, Jörg. 1995. "Die Indikationen zur Pränataldiagnostik müssen neu begründet werden" [The indications for prenatal diagnosticsmust be reestablished]. In Medizinische Genetik [Medical genetics] 1:49–52.

Schmidtke, Jörg, Brigitte Pabst, and Irmgard Nippert. 2005. "DNA-Based Genetic Testing Is Rising Steeply in a National Health Care System with Open Access to Services: A Survey of Genetic Test Use in Germany, 1996–2002." In Genetic Testing 9(1):80–84.

Schwarz, Clarissa M., and Beate Schücking. 2004. "Adieu, normale Geburt? Ergebnisse eines Forschungsprojektes" [Adieu, normal birth? Results of a research project]. In Dr.med.Mabuse 148:22–25.

Selting, Margaret. 1998. "Gesprächsanalytisches Transkriptionssystem (GAT)" [Transcription system for conversation analysis]. In Linguistische Berichte [Linguistic reports] 173:91–122.

Taylor, Janelle S. 2000. "Of Sonograms and Baby Prams: Prenatal Diagnosis, Pregnancy, and Consumption." Feminist Studies 26(2):391–418.

Theile, Ursel. 1977. Genetische Beratung: Motivationsanalyse [Genetic counseling: Motivation analysis]. München: Urban & Schwarzenberg.

Waldschmidt, Anne. 1996. Das Subjekt in der Humangenetik: Expertendiskurse zur Programmatik und Konzeption der genetischen Beratung, 1945–1990 [The subject in human genetics: Expert discourses on the objectives and conceptual design of genetic counseling, 1945–1990]. Münster: Westfälisches Dampfboot.

Watkins, Elizabeth Siegel. 1998. On the Pill: A Social History of Oral Contraceptives, 1950–1970. Baltimore: Johns Hopkins University Press.
Wendt, Gerhard G. 1975. Erbkrankheiten: Risiko und Verhütung [Hereditary diseases: Risk and prevention]. Marburg: Die Medizinische Verlagsgesellschaft.
Wertz, Dorothy C., and John C. Fletcher. 2004. Genetics and Ethics in Global Perspective. Dordrecht: Kluwer Academic.
Weß, Ludger, ed. 1989. Die Träume der Genetik: Gentechnische Utopien von sozialem Fortschritt [The dreams of genetics: Genetic utopias of social progress]. Nördlingen: Greno.
Williams, Clare, Priscilla Alderson, and Bobbie Farsides. 2002. "Is Nondirectiveness Possible within the Context of Antenatal Screening and Testing?" In Social Science and Medicine 54(3):339–47.
Zerres, Klaus. 2003. "Humangenetische Beratung" [Genetic counseling]. In Deutsches Ärzteblatt [German medical journal] 100(42):A2720–A2727.
Zuuren, Florence J. van, E. C. M. van Schie, and N. K. van Baaren. 1997. "Uncertainty in the Information Provided during Genetic Counseling." In Patient Education and Counseling 32(1–2):129–39.

Shifting responsibilities in the medical field: US-American bioethics and its move into the hospital setting

HELEN KOHLEN

How bedside ethics gave way to bioethics is the subject matter of this article.[1] In this transformation process, the evolvement and development of institutionalized ethics committees have played a decisive role. They serve as a vehicle for the historical analysis. The driving forces that gave impetus for establishing these committees and the way they have been shaped by bioethics are identified. The key questions are: what are the driving forces behind calling upon experts of bioethics—sitting in hospital committees—and what are the consequences of collective decision-making and a rationalistic framework for resolving "patients' cases"?

Bioethics, understood as a contested discipline and practice whose historical traces and proper tasks are not clear at all, has nevertheless been growing as an interdisciplinary enterprise in the US since the 1960s. Bioethicists are called upon to serve as expert consultants in numerous medical, legal, political, educational and industrial areas. In the 1970s, the "Case of Karen Quinlan" drove the idea of decision-making by local committees

---

1 The work is based on the author's transnational research study about bioethics and hospital ethics committees in the US and Germany (2009). The findings are analyzed from a historically situated medical sociological perspective.

forward. Gradually, bioethics began moving into the medical field as ethics committees became the standardized organizational form for reviewing patient care and engaging in a collective decision-making process, formulating new rules and policies, and educating health care professionals about coping with ethical dilemmas.

Medical morality gave way to bioethics by adopting not only its interdisciplinary approach, but also its rational analytical style and a technical procedure of principle-based ethics. Hereby, the responsibility, which was once under the authority of the medical profession, rooted in the Hippocratic oath, began shifting into a collective decision-making process by a team of (bio-) ethics experts, physicians, lawyers, nurses, chaplains and social workers.

Since it was the duty of those in the medical field, generally it was the individual physician who read and wrote about moral matters like withholding a course of antibiotics from an elderly patient whose story and condition so indicates, and whose wish it is to die. Based on a relationship of trust, decision-making was assigned by proximity, that is to say, the physician knowing the patient and the situation decided on ethical questions at the bedside or in the privacy of the hospital room.

Since the 1960s US-American bioethics has been growing as an interdisciplinary enterprise that has gradually moved into the medical field. In the 1970s ethics committees such as research ethics committees and hospital ethics committees (HECs)[2] were established. While the first ones served to review medical research proposals, the second ones dealt with patient care review. By the end of the 1980s, HECs became standing committees resolving questions on withholding and withdrawing treatment from a gravely ill newborn or terminally ill adult. Both adopted the interdisciplinary approach of bioethics and made use of principle-based ethics.

Medical ethics began shifting its focus from care and responsibility to autonomy and justice. The responsibility, once under the authority of the medical profession, rooted in the Hippocratic oath, shifted into a collective decision-making process by a multidisciplinary team of (bio-)ethics experts, lawyers, nurses, chaplains and social workers. Both the style and substance of medical decision-making changed. Increasingly, formal discus-

---

2   Clinical ethics committees (CECs) and institutional ethics committees (IECs) are synonyms.

sions with patients and the attention of journalists, judges, or professional philosophers began to take place.

What bioethics is understood to be, when and why it was understood to evolve and develop, who plays a role, and what characterizes the bioethical language and framework are the questions dealt with in the first part of the analysis. How medical ethics at the bedside gave way to bioethics in the hospital setting will then be analyzed by focussing on the development of local hospital ethics committees. These committees are identified as a vehicle that brought the style and shape of bioethics into the hospital arena, affecting concrete medical practices. As an environment for analysis, the committees serve to see how the handling of principle-based ethics has shifted the perspectives of who is responsible for what and whom.

THE BIOETHICAL TURN INTO THE MEDICAL FIELD

For medical sociologists Renee Fox and Judith Swazey, who carried out one of the first critical analyses of the field of bioethics, the term "bioethics" came into use as a neologism in the 1960s "to refer to the rise of professional and public interest in moral, social, and religious issues connected with the 'new biology' and medicine and to the emergence of an interdisciplinary field of inquiry and action concerned with these issues" (Fox/Swazey 1984: 336).

While medical ethics is very much associated with professional obligations and responsibilities for patients in need of medical care, bioethics is much more difficult to grasp in the sense of who perform roles of responsibility and which activities are performed. In an article Medical Morality is Not Bioethics, Fox and Swazey (1984) started to investigate the phenomenon of bioethics by looking at its cultural and historical context of expansion. They question both the intellectual assumptions and the methods of bioethics. The authors criticize philosophers, explicitly Tristram Engelhardt, who announced himself to be a "bioethicist," for viewing bioethics as largely a-cultural and trans-cultural in nature. Fox later (1996) explains in her article More than Bioethics, that the expansionary use of the term ethics and bioethics is connected with a larger social phenomenon. She argues that US-American bioethics needs to be understood as an expression as well as a part of the society and culture from which it has evolved. She explains:

Bioethics is not, and never has been, 'just bioethics'... First, there has always been ambiguity about whether bioethics could or should be defined in strict disciplinary and academic terms. Although its founders and most prominent contributors have been highly trained in particular disciplines (pre-eminently philosophy, theology, the law, and medicine), from the outset of history, bioethics has been a multidisciplinary field, actively involved in clinical and policy application, as well as in reflection and inquiry, whose locus and outreach extend beyond the academy and professional enclaves into the public domain. Paradoxically, as bioethics has become more recognized and consolidated institutionally, the conception of the field, of its orbit, and of its practitioners has become more diffuse and imprecise (Fox 1996: 6).

A relation between the flourishing of bioethics and a growing public suspicion of medicine has also been discussed. The use of an ethical profession found within the discipline of bioethics is interpreted as an answer to this suspicion (DeVries/Conrad 1998: 240). In sum, bioethics is considered to be influenced by the following triad: individualism, pluralism, secularization:

Because secularised society lacks a foundation for ethical decision-making, moral dilemmas, once readily solved with reference to a faith tradition, now require the articulation of nonreligious solutions. Pluralism demands arbitration between cultures—a niche neatly filled by a bioethicist. And the rise of individualism ... diminishes the role of community in ethical decision-making, creating a need for ethical guidance. (DeVries/Conrad 1998: 240)

The authors pinpoint these characteristics back to the 1960s, when agitation over civil rights, the Vietnam War, as well as issues of women's liberation led to widespread questioning of institutional authority and an ambition to handle structural injustice. According to their analysis, the occupational world was the one supporting the growing specialty of bioethics at that time (DeVries/Conrad 1998: 240). They argue: "More specifically, medicine, an occupation fragmented into many specialties, was (and is) organizationally prepared to accept an ethical specialist." (DeVries/Conrad 1998: 241) The dynamics created by a combination of these conditions prepared the ground for the development of bioethics.

Turning to the issues discussed in the field of bioethics, the questions arise: What is considered to be a bioethical concern worth dealing with?

What is not defined as a bioethical problem and therefore not dealt with? How are the issues framed? What kind of thinking is emphasized? Who participates in the field of bioethics and what kind of language is used?

Since the 1960s, bioethics has primarily been concerned with issues associated with technological progress (Stevens 2000), and not with the promises it holds forth, such as anticipated developments in genetic screening and counselling, birth technology, artificial kidney machines, life support systems, and organ transplantation. Furthermore, bioethics has also been dealing with the proper definition of life and death as well as personhood. In the clinical arena, another dominantly discussed issued has been the justifiability of foregoing life-sustaining forms of medical therapy. One of the most evolving general characteristics of the ensemble of concerns is that they all cluster, at least to some degree, around problems of natality and mortality, questions surrounding the beginning and the end of human life.

Since the mid-1970s another issue being considered bioethical is the allocation of scarce, expensive resources for advanced medical care, research and development. Fox and Swazey critically explain:

The resources with which bioethics is chiefly concerned are material ones, mainly economic and technological in nature. The allocation of nonmaterial resources such as personnel, talent, skill, time, energy, caring, and compassion is rarely mentioned. Bioethics situates its allocation questions within a rather abstract, individual rights-oriented notion of the general or common good, assigning greater importance to equity than to equality. The ideally moral distribution of goods is defined as one that all rational, self-interested persons are willing to accept as just and fair, even if goods are allotted unequally. (Fox/Swazey 1984: 353)

Absent in bioethical deliberations about risk pools and managed care organizations (MCOs) is a consideration of the administrative costs of these organizations.

Although in bioethics literature one can generally find the explanation that new medical and technological advances drive bioethics to provide answers to questions about values, Raymond DeVries and Peter Conrad declare this technologically-bound explanation to be empirically false (DeVries/Conrad 1998: 240). Questions generated by new technology, they state, are not new ones. Advances in medical technology, the issues of euthanasia, withholding or withdrawing treatment, truth telling, informed consent, as well as equitable access to health care have existed a long time. On the contrary, medical science has been introducing new machines and new techniques regularly over the past century and many of these have reframed the moral questions of medicine. What is new, is making these concerns a public issue. And why call for a bioethical specialist? The presence of technology had not necessarily called for a bioethical specialist since several existing occupations could have been asked, such as lawyers, clergy and social workers who routinely give counsel in matters of life and death and were available to give counsel on the use of new technology in the 1960s and 1970s (DeVries/Conrad 1998: 240).

The emphasis bioethics had placed on individualism and contractual relations ended up downplaying and obscuring the interconnectedness of persons and thus minimizing the social as well as moral importance of their interrelatedness (Fox/Swazey 1984: 354). It struck Fox that voices of venerated figures like Paul Ramsey's and Hans Jonas's were rare among bioethicists. Questions of social conscience and responsibility had little influence on the master conceptual framework of the field of "the principalism of analytic philosophy" (Fox 1996: 6). The dominance of the principle of autonomy in Anglo-American analytic philosophy grew into the regnant intellectual framework of American bioethical thought. Fox and Swazey explain:

… it is the individual, seen as an autonomous, self-determining entity rather than in relationship to significant others, that is the starting point and the foundation stone of American bioethics. Herein lie some of the deepest intellectual and philosophical difficulties that we have experienced as two of the relatively few social scientists who have been professionally associated with bioethics since its inception (Fox/Swazey 1984: 229).

How did principle-based ethics begin? First, it was the Belmont report that started out with a principle-based ethics to review and regulate research in the medical field. The Belmont report was issued in 1979 by the National Commission and defined three principles: respect for persons, beneficence, and justice (Moreno 1995: 76). These principles aimed at providing an analytical framework guiding the resolution of ethical problems arising from research on human subjects. In order to evaluate the acceptability of medical research with patients of health care institutions, the establishment of institutional review boards (IRBs) was mandated. From the movement toward IRBs, in general, Jonathan Moreno sees an appreciation at the federal level "that decisions concerning human beings in research are not only purely scientific matters, but also they involve the consideration of moral values" (Moreno 1995: 97). The establishment of IRBs is distinctive in that it led to statutory requirements for an ethics committee review of processes which would formerly have been regarded strictly a matter of professional competence. As a significant fact, Moreno stresses that specific standards of judgement are imposed on all such bodies in the form of ethical principles (Moreno 1995: 98).

Beyond medical research, the climax of rationalistic, principle-based medical ethics in the practical arena began with the first publication of Beauchamp and Childress' Principles of Biomedical Ethics (1983). Major territorial claims for the basic principles were mapped out during the late 1970s and dominated the discussion of medical ethics during the 1980s. "The problem of relying overly much on principles in medical ethics is that agreement on principles may not lead to agreement on conclusions, and agreement on conclusion may not imply an agreement on principles" (Thomasma 1994: 88). When a protest developed on the essential tidiness of an ethics of principles, it centered largely on an overreliance on the principle of autonomy. This led to an analysis of the strengths and weaknesses of an autonomy-based medical ethics. One weakness identified was that it would leave out "the essential partner in the medical encounter, the physician" (Pellegrino/Thomasma 1988).

In the 1980s, critical reviews of bioethics as well as self-criticism[3] started to be discussed. Fox observed that most philosophers in the field of bioethics contended that the triumph of the principle of autonomy was essential for general and medical reasons. The key subject of the criticism was not how to get rid of autonomy, but how to prevent it from receiving such moral focus. The question was: How can ignoring values above and

---

[3] Daniel Callahan for example, criticized too much emphasis on the language of rights of American individualism and of American courts (1980: 1230). In another article he points out that the principle of autonomy has been given an exaggerated importance whereas other values have not been sufficiently looked at (Callahan 1984: 42).

beyond autonomy be avoided, especially socially ethical ones? (Fox 1990: 211)[4] Fox resumes that the priority bioethics has accorded to individualism and its focus on autonomy had diverted its gaze from particular kinds of social issues that affect persons in society who are poor, discriminated against, and marginalized. And moreover, it had drawn lines between what are defined as social and as ethical matters (Fox 1996: 7). She recounts one of her most memorable examples of the tendency to separate the ethical from the social which occurred during her service on the President's Commission for the Study of Ethical Problems in Medicine and Biomedical and Behavioural Research from 1979 to 1982:

... a number of commissioners argued that although inequitable access to health care in the United States was a serious problem, and we had been mandated by Congress to study the ethical and legal implications of differences in the availability of health services as determined by income or residence of the person receiving the service, it was not a topic appropriate for our deliberations because it was a social issue, with policy and political implications, rather than an ethical one. After a period of intense negotiation, the Commission agreed to undertake the study, and to include race and ethical origins as additional factors to be examined in evaluating differences in the availability of health care. The result was the volume entitled Securing Access to Health Care, published in March 1983, with whose conclusions not all the members of the commission agreed (Fox 1996: 7).

From the outset, as the term "bio-ethics" as a compound noun denotes, a broad-based interdisciplinary approach was intended in which not only one discipline or discourse was to be dominant. Usually, areas of study have their own vocabulary, but characteristic for the field of bioethics is its conglomerated linguistic shape. The language of bioethics tends to be specifically eclectic, due to its development in an interdisciplinary setting and especially its acquisition of vocabulary from medicine, philosophy, theology, and law.

---

4   This concern was revealed in the Hastings Center's symposium on Autonomy, Paternalism, and Community to celebrate its fifteenth anniversary in 1984. Caution was expressed about an ethics that stresses individual autonomy while neglecting the obligation to the human community (Fox 1990: 211).

With regard to the participants in the field of bioethics, the main professional representatives in American bioethics have been philosophers, theologians—pre-dominantly Catholic and Protestant—, jurists, physicians, and biologists. In the 1980s, when allocation of so-called "scarce resources" and cost containment problems entered the field of bioethics, economists joined the group. Although bioethicists have considered macro-allocative problems in the sense of a fair distribution of medical services that tackles socio-political thoughts and the field of social science, relatively few social scientists have been actively involved or notably influential in bioethical debates. The limited participation of sociologists, political scientists and anthropologists in bioethics can be explained by a complex phenomenon:

... caused as much by the prevailing intellectual orientations and the weltanschauung of present-day American social science as by the framework of bioethics, ... the status and role of jurists in bioethics are integrally connected with the singular importance that Americans attach to the principle as well as to the fact of being 'a society under law, rather than under men'. (Fox/Swazey 1984: 350)

The struggle to find a proper, mutually agreeable way of organizing themselves in order to gain legitimacy and strength has been more challenging for bioethicists than their effort to find a proper intellectual framework (DeVries/Conrad 1998: 242). Fox and Swazey (1984) identify an overlap between the rationalism of American law, its emphasis on individual rights, and the ways in which it has been shaped by Western traditions of natural law, positivism, and utilitarianism, reinforcing key attributes of the philosophical thought in bioethics. The majority of the philosophers most active in bioethics were trained in analytical philosophy with an emphasis "on theory, methodology, and technique, ... utilitarian, neo-Kantian, and 'contractarian' outlooks" (Fox 1990: 208). The philosophical positivism is shaped by the scientific principles and rules that are well-known by biologists who have been educated to apply this style of scientific thinking to their work. Rigor, precision, clarity, consistency as well as objectivity are regarded as earmarks of an intellectually and ethically favourable kind of moral thought. This way of thinking tends toward dichotomous distinctions and bipolar choices:

Self versus others, body versus mind, individual versus group, public versus private, objective versus subjective, rational versus nonrational, lie versus truth, benefit versus harm, rights versus responsibilities, independence versus dependence, autonomy versus paternalism, liberty versus justice are among the primary ones. (Fox/Swazey 1984: 355).

In addition to analytical argumentation and a technical procedure of problem definition driven by the identification of ethical and legal principles, it is also applied pragmatism that has become influential in the medical field. Applied pragmatism of the bioethical framework contributes to the way in which problems are handled in the practical arena, for example in the hospital. Those involved, such as physicians, nurses, hospital administrators, patients, families, lawyers, politicians, and their associates are expected to decide what to do and what not to do in real-life (life and death) situations, and then not write or talk, but act on the ground of their determination and consensus (Fox 1990: 209).

Daniel Chambliss observed that the use of bioethical language in hospitals has first of all made moral debates more abstract by continually referring to general principles:

Left aside, often, are discussions of the general routines or structures of medical services. Such language is legalistic in tone and sometimes indistinguishable from legal advice. An 'ethics consultation' in American hospitals often includes the hospital lawyer, and decisions on what is right are regularly tempered by what the courts officially sanction as legal. Where the language of ethics frames debate, certain issues find no place in the conversation. At the same time, this language can be a weapon for those who know it. (Chambliss 1996: 4)

As pointed out by the findings of Fox and others, in the framework and language of bioethics, questions of autonomy rather than questions of responsibility are put forward. Where does this lead? Can questions of individual autonomy and justice grasp conflicts of concern in the practical arena of the hospital, especially when dealing with the most vulnerable and dependent people? In the following, the bioethical move into the hospital setting will be analyzed, seeing how its style, shape and language has influenced the work of ethics committees and changed ethical decision-making at the bedside.

BIOETHICS BY COMMITTEES

The move of bioethics into the hospital setting can be described as a move from the "periphery to the center" (Chambers 2000: 22). David Rothman explains:

It was usually the individual physician who decided .. matters at the bedside or in the privacy of the hospital room, without formal discussions with patients, their families, or even with colleagues, and certainly without drawing the attention of journalists, judges, or professional philosophers. And they made their decisions on a case-by-case basis, responding to the particular circumstances as they saw fit, reluctant to both training and practice to formulate or adhere to guidelines or rules. (Rothmann 2003: 2)

Rothman (2003) identifies bioethicists as "strangers at the bedside" since medical decision-making no longer lies in the authority of the physician. He explains: "By the mid-1970s, both the style and substance of medical decision-making had changed. The authority that an individual physician had once exercised covertly was now subject to debate and review by colleagues and laypeople." (Rothman 2003: 2) Bioethicists are called upon to serve as expert consultants in numerous medical, legal, political and educational fields, including the hospital arena. Because professional practitioners and policy makers feel overwhelmed with difficult questions, especially concerning end-of-life issues, they call upon so-called "bioethics experts", intellectuals and academics, expected to help resolve concrete problems in a reasonably clear way (Fox 1990: 209). Rothman describes the change in the following way:

Let the physician decide to withdraw or terminate life-sustaining treatment from an incompetent patient, and in the room were state judges to rule, in advance, on the legality of these actions. Such a decision might also bring into the room a hospital ethics committee staffed by an unusual cadre of commentators, the bioethicists, who stood ready to replace bedside ethics with armchair ethics, to draw on philosophers' first principles, not on the accumulated experience of medical practice. (Rothman 2003: 2)

The fact is that bioethicists are being asked to help professional practitioners and policymakers come up with specific ways of resolving concrete medical-moral problems. For Fox and Swazey, "this advisory role to decision makers has reinforced the cognitive predisposition of bioethics to distill the complexity and uncertainty, the dilemmas and the tragedy out of the situations they analyse ... (and this implies) a new, expedient justification for the forms of intellectual and moral reductionism in which it engages" (Fox/Swazey 1984: 358).

DeVries and Conrad think that bioethics has been successful in altering the behavior of physicians (DeVries/Conrad 1998: 245). They argue that bioethics in the clinical setting can enforce a moral 'deskilling' of physicians and other professionals. The decisions regarding responsibilities of care are transferred to bioethicists.

The role of a bioethicist "is much like that of a public defender in the American legal system. The formal role of each is to represent the interests of a client in a large and confusing bureaucracy, many of whom are working against the interest of their clients" (DeVries/Conrad 1998: 246). They conclude: "Given this organizational situation, bioethicists will be inclined to represent the interests of medical professionals and medical institutions over those who are merely passing through—patients and families" (DeVries/Conrad 1998: 246).

As already pointed out in the first part of this article, the shape of bioethics and its definition of problems exclude others, such as social and communal matters of concern. That this also accounts for the clinical setting is revealed by the following example, drawn from the context of the neonatal intensive care unit. Fox says that bioethical attention has been put on the

justifiability of non-treatment decisions, but relatively little attention has been paid to the fact that a disproportionately high number of extremely premature infants of very low birth weight, with severe congenital abnormalities, cared for in NICUs are babies born to poor, disadvantaged mothers, many of whom are single teenagers, and also nonwhite.(Fox 1990: 208)

Fox states: "these kinds of social problems are 'de-listed' as ethical problems in a manner that removes them from the sphere of moral scrutiny and concern." (Fox 1990: 208)

How can this system continue to function unaltered? Paul Wolpe (1998) argues that it is the individualistic stance of American bioethics that leaves the existing system unchallenged. Chambliss, Fox, DeVries and Conrad have observed that bioethicists ignore certain obvious questions about the structure of health care and this lack of sensitivity prevents American bioethicists from seeing the way they are protecting the status quo. The decade-long field study by Chambliss revealed:

Talk of 'ethical dilemmas' diverts attention from the structural conditions that have produced the problem in the first place. This is naturally in the interest of the status quo and is relatively unthreatening to powerful interests within the hospital. This is why so many hospitals can readily accept an 'ethics committee' and its debates about ethical issues. Initially, some powerful hospital staff may feel threatened, but the threat is contained by framing issues as 'difficult dilemmas' rather than seeing them as symptoms of the structural flaws of the health care system. (Chambliss 1996: 92-93)

Based on fieldwork, for Chambliss (1996: 3) it is clear that bioethicists as well as ethics committees serve the interest of medical organizations.

In 1976, the New Jersey Supreme Court's decision in the case of Karen Ann Quinlan was seen as crucial for certifying the legal right of formerly competent patients to refuse treatment. This decision heightened the topic of local ethics committees in the hospital for an interdisciplinary decision-making process. Rothman emphasizes:

The culmination of the decade-long process of bringing strangers to the bedside came in the case of Karen Quinlan. Its impact on opinion and policy outweighed even that of the scandals in human experimentation ... After Quinlan there was no disputing the fact that medical decision making was in the public domain and that a profession that had once ruled was now being ruled. (Rothman 2003: 222)

The license and corresponding responsibilities of deciding questions of life and death shifted from the profession to the polity, from the hospital intensive care unit and physicians' authority over ethics to the open courtroom and ethics committees. How did the story start and develop?

In April 1975 Karen Quinlan, at the age of twenty-two, was brought into a New Jersey hospital emergency room (Rothman 2003: 222). Though she was diagnosed irreversibly brain damaged and to be in a so-called "persistent vegetative state", she was not "brain-dead" and the etiology of her coma was never fully explained (Sichel 1992: 114). After several months of hope, her parents recognized that she would not recover and they asked her physicians to remove her from the respirator which had been assisting her breathing. Her mother, Julia and her father, Joseph Quinlan, practicing Catholics, were looking for church guidance and had been told that taking Karen off the machine, even if she would die then, was morally a correct action since this would return their daughter to her "natural state" whereas respiratory care was seen as "extraordinary" (Rothman 2003: 222). St. Clair's hospital staff initially responded to the parents' request to discontinue the treatment. The hospital made them sign a paper declaring that the responsible physician, Dr. Morse, was authorized and directed to discontinue all extraordinary measures, including the use of a respirator for Karen. The document noted that the physicians had explained all the consequences of the removal and the parents felt relieved, but not the physician: The next day, he called to tell them that he had a "moral problem" with the agreement, and that he intended to consult a colleague. When he called the day after, he informed them that he would not remove Karen from the respirator (Rothman 2003: 222-223). Rothman remarks:

The staff would not even consider removing Karen from the respirator unless a court formally appointed them Karen's legal guardians. ... Dr. Morse, and the other physicians who testified on his behalf, scrupulously differentiated between withholding treatment in the hopeless case, which was allowable, and withdrawing treatment from the hopeless case, which ostensibly was not. (Rothman 2003: 223-227)

The Quinlans went before the Superior Court of New Jersey to ask that the father be appointed Karen's guardian for the express purpose of requesting Karens' removal from the respirator (Rothman 2003: 224). In November 1975 the lower court rejected the petition. The hospital reserved judgement, because due to any criteria, including the Harvard brain-death standards, Karen was said to be alive, and disconnecting her from the respirator might well "open the doctors and the hospital to criminal prosecution for homicide" (Rothman 2003: 223). Betty Sichel is convinced:

The court justified its decision not to authorize removal of the respirator, noting that the rapid advancement of medical knowledge made it impossible to foresee what future knowledge would mean for the patient's health, recognizing the absence of medical tradition to warrant the act, and referring to legal precedent. (Sichel 1992: 114)

The parents then went before the State's Supreme Court which accepted the case. The justices wrestled with the question of whether or not Quinlan's respirator could be disconnected. The court finally accepted the lawyer's argument, that a "constitutionally protected right to privacy overlay the doctor-patient relationship" (Rothman 2003: 225).

And how did the court's decision affect the professional role of physicians? The end of the Karen Quinlan story raised the question, whether the court could dare to tell physicians how to treat, or not to treat, their patients. If the court could not be seen as the potentially right place to deal with difficult questions such as those brought up by the Quinlan story, what was the alternative? In order to deal with the burden of a physician's responsibility of deciding whether a patient should live or die, attention was increasingly drawn to collective decision-making by committees.

At the time when Karen Quinlan was raising widespread attention, New Jersey's justices were impressed by a Baylor Law Review article, written by a pediatrician named Karen Teel (1975). She inspired the proposal of a local committee in the case of Karen Quinlan "for more input and dialogue in individual situations and to allow the responsibility of these judgements to be shared". (Teel 1975: 9)[5] Teel contended that physicians are charged with the responsibility of making ethical judgements for which they are sometimes "ill-equipped" on intellectual grounds and "knowingly or not, (assume) civil and criminal liability" (Teel 1975: 8). The proposed multidisciplinary committee would not only bring a new and valuable dialogue to the medical decision-making process but from a legal point of view, share and divide responsibility (Teel 1975: 8). Although Teel saw such a committee as being "advisory" rather than "enforcing", the New Jersey court had given it a greater role. In their landmark decision they ruled that if Quinlan's attending physician determined that there was no "reasonable

---

5 There had been clinical ethics committees before official establishment as Teel points out in the article.

chance" that she would ever return to a "cognitive, sapient state," and if a hospital ethics committee agreed with that prognosis, then the life support apparatus could be withdrawn at her guardian's or family's request on the basis of an individual's right of privacy. With this sort of mechanism, the physician would be immune from civil or criminal liability (Cranford 1984:14). Recognizing that the constitutional right of privacy applied to the refusal of medical treatment, the court held the opinion that Karen Quinlan's right to privacy should not be surrendered because she was "incompetent" (Murphy 1989: 552).

The judge at the Supreme Court had understood something very different than Karen Teel had meant. Although the court had taken up her suggestion and called for a hospital ethics committee, as a way to serve and protect hospitals by reviewing the individual circumstances of the dilemma, to assist families and help physicians in reaching appropriate decisions, it did not show any interest in its multidisciplinary character: "The court's concept of an ethics committee was to consist wholly of physicians." (Moreno 1995: 98) Their assumption of where to settle an "ethical dilemma" was made on the basis of medical descriptions and definitions and charged it to decide no other issues of a case, but the narrower technical questions of whether the patient was in a chronic "vegetative state" or whether any "reasonable" chance of recovery existed (Rothman 2003: 228). As noted by Norman Fost and Ronald E. Cranford the expression "hospital ethics committee" in this case was a misnomer since their real intention was to obtain a neurological diagnosis given by medical experts (Fost/Cranford 1985: 2688).

Although talk about ethics committees subsided after the Quinlan case, in many hospitals, doctors, nurses, hospital administrators, and social workers started meeting regularly in small groups, called for example, "bioethics study groups", to discuss clinical problems they were facing and began to regularly organize meetings for a shared decision-making process. In an expert interview (Kohlen 2009: 72) Ruth Purtillo, who describes herself as being a "part of the history of bioethics", explains: "After some time, they took on a more formal role in the hospital and began to provide education programs within the institution and worked on guidelines that would help to make decision making less traumatic" (Kohlen 2009: 72-73). In the 1970s, two hospitals in Boston, Massachusetts (Massachusetts General Hospital and Beth Israel Hospital) and one health care institution in

New York (Montefiore Medical Center), ranked among the first to describe the formation and work of their committees. David Rothman refers especially to the formation of a committee in Massachusetts General Hospital (MGH) by explaining:

With public scrutiny heightened, a few hospitals took steps to bring greater formality to the decision-making process. The Quinlan decision became the occasion for setting up committees to advise and review termination decisions and to formulate guidelines for individual physicians. Thus, the Massachusetts General Hospital administrators appointed an ad hoc committee to study 'how best to manage the hopelessly ill patient. (Rothman 2003: 229)

It was at the beginning of the 1970s when MGH administrators appointed a psychiatrist, two physicians, a nursing administrator, a layperson and "legal counsel" to an ad hoc committee. A classification system was recommended, especially for patients with brain death or when there was no reasonable possibility that the patient would regain a cognitive and sapient life. This four-point patient-classification system, then established by MHG, ranged from A: meaning "maximal therapeutic effort without reservation" to D: meaning "all therapy can be discontinued" (Rothman 2003: 229). In 1974 Boston Massachusetts Hospital turned its ad-hoc-committee into an institutional ethics committee, called the Optimum Care Committee (OCC). The management of end-of-life care was its main task. They dealt with intervention "in situations where difficulties arise in deciding the appropriateness of continuing intensive therapy for critically ill patients" (Rothman 2003: 230). The members were a surgeon, an internist who was also a lawyer, and the chairperson, a psychiatrist with a divinity degree. First, the committee only met at the request of the attending physician who needed to record the prognosis for the patient. Then, the committee role was advisory: its members consulted with one another, sometimes as a group and sometimes by telephone, and discussed the case. "They are guided mainly by a principle of beneficence, asking what would be the best thing to do for the patient." (Brennan 1988: 803) The completed recommendation went back to the physician, who was free to accept or reject its advice.

1974 through 1986, the committee's seventy-three consultations represented a wide range of experience with the problems arising when care for terminally ill patients was limited. Brennan, a committee participant, evaluates the collected data in an article Ethics Committees and Decisions to Limit Care. The Experience at the Massachusetts General Hospital (1988). It appeared that more families had been requesting the withdrawal of care when there was no hope of recovery. Many physicians hesitated to defer to the family's wish that mechanical ventilatory support or hydration be stopped. In numerous cases there were either no family, or the family members were far away and would not make a decision for their relative. In other situations the family was divided, and some families did not want limitations on care despite the fact that the patient was clearly not going to recover (Brennan 1988: 806). However, the court deferred judgement on issue of DNR (Do Not Resuscitate) status when the family and the physician disagreed (Brennan 1988: 807). Brennan remarks:

the role of ethics committees in making these decisions is not clear. It is not easy to say whether an ethics committee should recommend that physicians overrule family wishes on the assumption that a rational person would opt for DNR status if terminally ill and incompetent. (Brennan 1988: 807)

Finally, after ten years of committee experience, Brennan is convinced of the idea of collective decision-making. His argument:

The experience of the OCC at the Massachusetts General Hospital is valuable because it provides a model for an ethics committee's role in limited care cases and highlights the questions that arise in such cases. No one person can provide answers to these questions. Rather, they must be addressed by ethicists, lawyers, judges, physicians, and thoughtful members of our society... the issues do not belong to the 'silent world' of physicians and patients and should be widely debated. (Brennan 1988: 807)

The Beth Israel Hospital referred to Quinlan and drew up guidelines for ordering a DNR code for a patient.

When a physician believed a patient to be 'irreversibly and irreparably ill,' with death 'imminent' (that is, likely to occur within two weeks), the physician could elect to discuss with an ad hoc committee, composed exclusively of doctors, whether death was so certain that resuscitation would serve no purpose. If the committee members unanimously agreed, and the competent patient made it his or her 'informed choice', then a DNR order would be entered in the patient's chart; should the patient be incompetent, the physician was to obtain the approval of the family and then enter the order. (Rothman 2003: 230)

These measures, despite being legally justified, were easily accepted, drew attacks and remained an exception: they were implemented with great caution and not readily adopted in other settings. Most hospitals did not adopt guidelines and resisted establishing committees.

In 1977, a committee, called the "Bioethics Committee" was formed at the Montefiore Medical Center in New York and served primarily as an educational, policy-making, as well as guideline-writing consultative committee "responsible directly to the president of the medical center" (Rosner 1985: 2694). During the same time period, the Hastings Center held a two-day conference on hospital ethics committees. Robert Veatch assessed the role of the committees and came to differentiate between four types: (1) committees reviewing ethical and other values in individual patient care decisions, (2) committees making more extensive ethical and policy decisions, (3) counselling committees, and (4) prognosis committees (Veatch 1977).

When the mandate of the National Commission for the Protection of Human Subjects was about to expire in 1978, it was transformed into the President's Commission for the Study of Ethical Problems in Medicine and Medical and Bio-behavioural Research (hereafter the President's Commission). The US Congress charged the Commission to provide a temporary, national body that would consider the problematic situations that had arisen in medicine primarily, but not exclusively, as a result of advances in medical technology (Ross 1986: 18-19; Rothman 2003: 189). The 10-person, multidisciplinary commission was chaired by an attorney (Morris Abrams) and began its work in 1980. Compared to the National Commission for the Protection of Human Subjects its mandate was broader and not confined to ethical questions in research. It was invited to alter or add to a list of issues. Like before, the commission studied the problems they addressed, listened to the specialists who helped them to think about the issues and withdrew in order to reflect on the questions from their own point of views. It then collaborated with the National Institute of Health's Office for Protection from Research Risks as well as the Food and Drug Administration in order to develop a guidebook for Institutional Review Boards. Based on the work that had been done in the 1960s and 1970s, the President's Commission identified consensus, disagreements and uncertainties. These were documented, and during its three-year tenure, the commission held public readings throughout the country, commissioned research studies and published nine reports on "medical-legal-ethical issues that seemed most pressing" (Ross 1986: 19). The reports provide practical decision-making policies, principles and guidelines. The most cited ones are: the Definition of Death, Informed Consent, Deciding to Forego Life-Sustaining Treatment, Screening, Counselling for Genetic Conditions, Genetic Engineering as well as Access to Health Care. The report Deciding to Forego Life-Sustaining Treatment is generally concerned with treatment decisions for incompetent patients. Permanently unconscious patients, seriously ill newborns as well as decisions about cardiopulmonary resuscitation and do-not-resuscitate orders are discussed in particular. Besides an analysis of the problems, the report includes specific recommendations and conclusions about who should make decisions to forego treatment and how those decisions should be made (President's Commission 1983).

A number of these reports have had considerable influence on public opinion and public policy, medical and hospital practice as well as legislative action, and legal decision-making. Fox supposes that the Commission's volumes on Defining Death (July 1981) and Deciding to Forego Life-Sustaining Treatment (March 1983) have probably had the most influence (Fox 1990: 205). Effect at a judiciary level is also stated by Ross: "court decisions routinely cite these reports as authoritative statements on bioethics issues" (Ross 1986: 19). Although the commission's recommendations did not have the force of law, they were embraced by courts and legislature and treated like unwritten laws.

The President's Commission concluded that in order to protect the interests of patients who lack decision-making capacity and to ensure their well-being and self-determination, health care staff along with administrators and trustees ought to explore and evaluate various formal and informal administrative arrangements for review and consultation, such as ethics committees, especially for decisions having life-or-death consequences. The commissioners realized the ongoing ethical problems in these decisions and suggested that hospitals themselves work out procedures in order to enhance decision making for "incompetent patients." Organized interdisciplinary forums were supposed to be a reasonable means of promoting collective decision-making processes. Ross recommends that hospital ethics committees be particularly familiar with the reports on (1) Defining Death and (2) Deciding to Forego Life-Sustaining Treatment as well as (3) Making Health Care Decisions and (4) Security Access to Health Care (Ross 1986:19). In the second report named above, the President's Commission recommends five possible roles for hospital ethics committees: (a) diagnostic and prognostic review; (b) staff education by providing forums for the discussion of ethical issues and methodological instruction in resolving ethical dilemmas; (c) institutional policy and guideline formulation with regard to specific ethical issues; (d) review of treatment decisions made by physicians, patients or surrogate; and (e) decision-making in specific cases. With respect to the educational task of hospital ethics committees, the Commission stresses the importance of diverse membership and shared perspectives. The committee should "... serve as a focus for community discussion and education." (President's Commission 1983: 160-163). According to the President's Commission, courts should only be used as decision-makers as a last resort. There was hope that hospital ethics committees would develop an ability to facilitate local, consensual decision-making.

Moreno criticizes the President's Commission's remarks on ethics committees in Deciding to Forego Life-Sustaining Treatment for its ambiguous treatment of committees as decision-makers (Moreno 1995: 100): on the one hand a decision-making role is strongly suggested and on the other hand the report declares that "no decisions" are to be made (President's Commission 1983: 163; Cranford/Doudera 1984: 13). Instead of having the doctor who takes complete responsibility for patients in these critical situations, the report supports the idea of having an institutional body to represent and safeguard the patient's interests.

Did the support of the idea of hospital ethics committees please physicians? "It is well known that many physicians are indifferent to, and frequently hostile to, what they regard as the 'intrusion' of ethics on their turf" (McCormick 1984: 153). Nevertheless, only a few physicians have raised strong voices against these committees. Jonathan Moreno explains:

My impression is that the Commission intended to allow the possibility that ethics committees could actually make decisions for specific patients when the only other option is going to court ... The most likely situation in which there would be a stark choice between a court and the ethics committee is that of a terminally ill and incapacitated patient lacking directives or a surrogate. (Moreno 1995: 100)

In 1983 the first national conference on hospital ethics committees was held in Washington DC. Problems regarding their composition, goals, functioning, scope of responsibility, mandate as well as financing were discussed (Rosner 1985: 2697). Whether decisions of ethics committees should be binding and whether an ethics committee should ever go to court to seek enforcement of its views were among the crucial questions being debated (Rosner 1985: 2697). In that year, the President's Commission cited a proposed model for establishing hospital ethics committees: the scope of authority of such committees would be to review treatment decisions made on behalf of "terminally ill incompetent patients, who request committee review, review medical decisions having ethical implications, provide counselling, establish guidelines, and educate" (Rosner 1985: 2696). The model bill also suggested multidisciplinary membership of nine persons appointed by the chief hospital administrators for one-year renewable terms (Rosner 1985: 2696).

While the President's Commission supported the building of hospital ethics committees, still another regulatory impetus for collective decision-making by ethics committees appeared shortly after the commission's reports: the Baby Jane Doe and Baby Doe cases. In spring 1982, a Down's syndrome child (Baby Jane Doe) with a malformed gullet was born in Bloomington, Indiana. Some physicians recommended immediate surgery while others thought that the infant's quality of life would not be good after treatment and therefore no operation should be performed. The baby should just be kept comfortable and allowed to die. The parents decided for non-treatment and the hospital administration went to court to reverse the parents' decision. During a series of court hearings, rulings, and appeals, the baby died of starvation. As long as recommendation was given by a physician, Indiana judges affirmed the parent's right to choose non-treatment for the child (Cranford 1984: 12-13).

The case received widespread and mostly negative publicity. Public outcry was reported in numerous newspapers, magazine articles and editorials, and a response to this highly publicized case was federal government intervention: the Department of Health and Human Services (DHHS) published regulations on neonatal care (Cranford 1984: 13). Health care professionals asked themselves how to avoid federal intervention, and as a consequence, the American Academy of Pediatrics promulgated policy on critically ill newborns in response to the proposed Baby Doe governmental regulations that had been finally struck down in court (Moreno 1995: 81). The Academy included recommendations for the formation of Infant Bioethical Review Committees that the DHHS's final rule acknowledged and strongly encouraged, but did not mandate its use in hospitals caring for newborns (McCormick 1984: 150).

In fall 1983, a baby was born with spina bifida and hydrocephaly in New York ("the case of Baby Doe"). The parents decided for conservative treatment and refused surgery. Parents and physicians risked legal involvement when treatment decisions were made in these "gray" areas, especially when life-prolonging or aggressive treatment was withheld.

Then in 1984, Federal Child Abuse Amendments plus the DHHS regulations required all states to have a mechanism for ensuring that their intensive care nurseries were not engaging in discriminatory practices and recommended using Infant Care Review Committees to review decisions on forgoing life-saving treatment for newborns as a less intrusive alternative to federal investigation. At the national level, the American Hospital Association and the Catholic Hospital Association declared formal recommendation about hospital ethics committees, seen as a potential means of ensuring good decision-making practices. Finally, even the American Medical Association began supporting ethics committees (Ross 1986: 7).

By early 1985 a survey had shown: among hospitals with neonatal intensive care units, more than half had ethics committees. A majority of teaching hospitals had ethics committees and it was discovered that even hospitals without ethics committees were considering forming them. By size, only hospitals with 500 beds or more showed a significant increase. Most commonly, administrators, nurses, and the clergy were found on the committee, followed by legal counsel, social workers, patient representatives, and philosopher ethicists. These committees facilitated decision-making by clarifying important issues, providing legal protection for hospital administration and staff, and making consistent hospital policies. (Cranford/Doudera 1984: 15)

In addition to court cases and government intervention, other conditions during the late 1970s and early 1980s fostered the belief that hospital ethics committees could resolve new and complex health care ethical dilemmas.

Firstly, the argument that new medical technology had been creating ethical situations persisted, and secondly, the argument was raised that patients and their relatives would no longer accept passive roles, but demanded an active part in making decisions about treatment. It resulted in the assumption that each human being is an autonomous agent who is capable of making decisions as long as being fully informed with regard to medical care and his or her life. Closely connected to this movement was the change of society's trust in physicians' behaviour (Rothman 2003: 222). Sichel points to questions of mistrust and thinks:

> malpractice suits against hospitals and physicians have caused health care professionals and institutions considerable concern about how they might protect themselves (and) ... time was ripe for a new structure for making medical ethical decisions an autonomous physician no longer could make all medical and ethical judgements for his or her patients. (Sichel 1992: 116)

Ross explains, that there was continuing hope that ethics committees could help health care providers and patients "find their way out of the maze created by modern, technological medicine" (Ross 1986: 7).

Both, the DHHS as well as the American Academy of Pediatrics strongly recommended that each hospital providing newborn care—especially the ones with neonatal intensive care units —form Infant Review Committees. The recommendations given by the Academy of Pediatrics and the DHHS could supplement the statement by the President's Commission that had endorsed the idea of ethics committees in general. Some state legislatures, hospitals and state medical associations as well as insurance companies passed resolutions that approved hospital ethics committees.

On the whole, Cranford and Doudera are convinced that the most compelling impetus has been the regulations—first given by government and then by professional organizations—as a reaction to the story of "Infant Doe", a case of non-treatment of a newborn with Down's syndrome (Cranford/Doudera 1984: 13). Following Judith Ross, ethics committees were at a crucial point since they had been given institutional support as well as governmental encouragement, but what they ought to do and the way they should do it had not been made precisely clear. Education, policy development and case review are said to be their potential functions:

They will need to define their own tasks carefully and to use their limited time and energy wisely ... must be able to bend their differences to find consensus, and yet preserve those differences so that they do not become rubber stamps for a single point of view. (Ross 1986: 8)

Although seldom referred to in the literature, noteworthy is that the impetus for ethics committees in the years following the court cases not only came from the government but also from self-regulation in the health care industry: mainly in the context of "quality assurance".

A 1992 action by the Joint Commission for the Accreditation of Healthcare Organizations (JCAHO) formalized the institutionalization of clinical ethics. For accreditation, hospitals and other health care institutions were required to have a mechanism in place "for the consideration of ethical issues arising in the care of patients" and to provide education to caregivers and patients on ethical issues in health care (JCAHO 1992: 105). Hospital ethics committees became the favoured way for institutions to respond to various new guidelines and requirements that should assure quality in hospitals (Tulsky/Fox 1996).

The state of New York, being oriented towards activism and regulations, requires ethics committees in every hospital and nursing home. Moreover, there are additional requirements and recommendations put forward by the Governor's Task Force on Life and the Law concerning decision-making on behalf of incapacitated patients without advance directives or a durable power of attorney for health care (Moreno 1995:102).

In 1992 the Task Force proposed that family members or close friends be legally recognized as surrogates for patients. "To provide some public assurance and accountability that surrogates are acting in good faith, all decisions to forego life-sustaining treatment for non-dying patients would be subject to retrospective review by a facility-based 'bioethics committee'" (Moreno 1995:102). The structure as well as general procedures including multidisciplinary membership were also set forth in the bill. If patients do not have a surrogate, the ethics committee itself was authorized to make decisions concerning the termination of life-sustaining treatment (Moreno 1995:102).

With the New York proposal, the history of ethics committees had reached the point of legally required procedural decision-making in the clinical setting. The task force hoped that bioethics committees would become accepted in analogy to institutional review boards (Moreno 1995: 103). "Once created by the medical profession as a consultative mechanism composed entirely of physicians, committees that took a role in clinical ethics review have gradually acquired more regulatory authority." (Moreno 1995: 103) In 1996, the American Society for Bioethics Consultation together with the American Society for Health and Human Values created a joint task force to explore standards for ethics consultation. After two years of meeting, drafting and revising documents, the results, called core competencies for health care ethics consultation was published in 1998 by the American Society for Bioethics and Humanities (Aulislo/Arnold/Youngner 1999). In 2003 at the first international assessment summit on hospital ethics committees, Cranford, who had been watching the development of ethics consultation in the United States, described that the most controversial issues of committee discussions were DNR, brain death, nutrition and hydration (Cranford 2002: 1).

From the 1980s on, critical considerations about the use of abstract principles in the practical arena have been raised. For example, questions of decision-making for "not-capacitated" patients would be often framed in terms of who decides for the patients. The debate then, Virginia Warren remarks, is on the question of authority (Warren 1992: 36-38). She also suggests that important aspects of the moral context are obscured by appeals for neutrality. By stressing the value of neutrality, particular features of the situation would often be ignored. For her, the dominant trend in philosophical ethics has been to regard people as best able to decide what is moral when least tied to place and time and when least bound by ties or partiality to family and community (Warren 1992: 36-38). This practice of abstracting oneself from the particularities produces two kinds of distortions: First, it denies consideration of those experiences that shape how an agent perceives their role in a situation. "By subtracting those features that shed light on their experience and life, such individuals may become, at least in part, invisible to themselves." (Warren 1992: 33) Second, distortion arises from the creation of and emphasis on a picture of "generic persons and relationships" (Warren 1992: 33). Hence, it is likely to lose important factors about psychological well-being, as well as other facets of character that have bearing on a particular situation or potential resolution.

With a focus on how case discussions are framed in clinical ethics, Patricia Flynn observed that the speakers are more concerned with ethical principles than the processes by which decisions can be reached. Negotiation took place, but there were no equal resources or equal power relationships in the organization or in the committee meetings (Flynn 1991: 183). She discovered that there is a pattern of talking in hospital ethics committees, when

... dealt with ethics at all was to present the case, and then someone would say: 'What is the ethical principle?' and another person, often the ethicist, would say, as in a mantra, 'autonomy' or 'allocation of resources'. The incantations of justice, autonomy, beneficence, non-maleficence, veracity, and fidelity were heard throughout the committees. In one committee, the chair would press for two ethical principles that were in conflict, so that the response might be, for example: 'autonomy' and he would ask 'versus?' and someone would sing out 'justice'. (Flynn 1991: 182)

As her report shows, an instrumental use of abstract principles comparable to machinery work evolves. Margaret Urban Walker critically asks:

Aren't abstract principles often given (sometimes new) meaning under the impact of concrete cases, rather than cases being simply 'decided' by the 'application' of principles? And who or what decides what is a 'case'—a moral problem—in the first place, as well what sort of case-subject to what principle or principles—it is? (Walker 1993: 34)

Walker is convinced that "a story, or better, history is the basic form of representation for moral problems" (Walker 1993: 35). Therefore, she suggests to ask "who the parties are, how they understand themselves and each other, what terms of relationship have brought them to this ... problematic point, and perhaps what social or institutional frames shape or circumscribe their options" (Walker 1993: 35). She states:

If moral accounts must make sense to those by whom, to whom, and about whom they are given, the integrity of these accounts is compromised when some parties to a moral situation are not heard or represented. If chances are missed for different perspectives that open critical opportunities, moral community is doubly ill served, alternate narratives go unexplored, and some members are in practice disqualified as agents of value. (Walker 1993:37)

It sounds like an engineering model that supports a technical way of dealing with "cases" and framing questions. Likewise, John Evans criticizes the use of principles as a method that takes the complexity of moral life actually lived and translates this information into scales by discarding information that resists translation and thus creates a language that brings order to difficult problems. He thinks that the principles were created to "enhance calculability and simplify bioethical decision–making" (Evans 2000: 32).

Conclusions

Analysis of the evolvement of bioethics reveals that there are different opinions on the origins of the field and role of bioethics and that the emergence cannot be reduced to technological progress. Bioethics as an interdisciplinary enterprise has contributed to a lack of clarity due to a melange of language. This ambiguous framework of bioethics has found its way into the practical arena of hospitals and is acted out in institutionalized ethics committees.

In the US, these hospital committees are embedded within and have taken their direction from the emergent discipline of bioethics. Consequently, some of the first initiatives took on the name "bioethics" by calling themselves "bioethics study groups" or "bioethics committees". The demand for an organized meeting place for case deliberations grew out of a complex interplay of events as well as intervention by the government and health care industry. The Quinlan story gave its first rise to hospital ethics committees, supported by the law: the committee was charged with making a medical determination that confirmed the attending physician's prognosis that Karen Quinlan would not return to a "cognitive state". Thus, the committee function initially turned out to be medical, and not ethical. The President's Commission encouraged shared decision-making by local committees, seeing it as a responsibility of the hospital institution. In the Infant Doe Regulations the DHHS expressed their conviction about committees reviewing difficult questions about neo-natal care. Finally, the statutory authority of ethics committees in the hospital arena was pushed by defining its existence as a point of quality assurance and criteria for hospital accreditation. As exemplified by the Optimum Care Committee in Boston Massachusetts General Hospital, questions about living and dying mainly end up in classification systems and the formulation of DNR orders, dictating decision-making at the bedside.

The language in hospital committees' "case discussions" is based on the vocabulary of principle-based ethics, used in a pragmatic way that had once proved to be helpful in dealing with ethical questions of research. While questions of autonomy and justice dominate, questions of responsibility are rather left out. Responsibilities are not clear, but who is responsible for whom, what, when and why do shift and can transfuse within the interdisciplinary discussions. It is a challenge to resist the principle-based model since its use can be time-saving and makes those participating feel safe by following a structure of "case analysis" that resembles the logic of law. The clarity helps to abstract from concrete persons who are often in situations that are on the contrary not clear at all. The use of principles helps to calculate and simplify decision-making processes. Instead, from a sociological and feminist philosophers point of view, narrative and history are essential in representing moral problems and social conflicts.

In sum, those currently taking on the work of ethics committees might benefit by reflecting critically upon the shape it has adopted from US American bioethics and raise questions about the way principle-based ethics is used. Elaborately technical means of collective ethical decision eclipse professional competencies of touch, truth and trust. The importance of clinical experience and practices of responsibility are at stake.

REFERENCES

Aulislo, Mark P./Arnold, Robert M./Youngner, Stuart J. (1999): "An ongoing conversation. The task force re-port and bioethics consultation", in: The Journal of Clinical Ethics 10(1), pp. 3-4.

Beauchamp, Tom/Childress, James F. (1983): Principles of biomedical ethics, 2nd edition. New York.

Brennan, Troyen A. (1988): "Ethics committees and decisions to limit care. The experience at the Massachusetts General Hospital", in: Journal of the American Medical Association (6), pp. 803-807.

Callahan, Daniel (1980): "Contemporary biomedical ethics", in: The New England Journal of Medicine 302, pp. 1228-1233.

— (1984): "Autonomy: A moral good, not a moral obsession", in: Hastings Center Report 14(5), pp. 40-42.

Chambers, Tod (2000): "Centering bioethics", in: Hastings Center Report 30(1), pp. 22-29.

Chambliss, Daniel F. (1996): Beyond caring. Hospitals, nurses, and the social organization of ethics, Chicago: Chicago University Press.

Cranford, Ronald E. (2002): The history of ethics consultation in the United States; http:/clevelandclinic.org/bioethics/cec/plenary_cranford.htm (last accessed 4/25/05).

Cranford, Ronald E./Doudera, A. E. (1984): "The emergence of institutional ethics committees", in: Law, Medicine & Ethics 12(1), pp. 13-20.

DeVries, Raymond/Conrad, Peter (1998): Why bioethics needs sociology, in: DeVries, Raymond/Subedi, Janardan (eds): Bioethics and society. Constructing the ethical enterprise, New Jersey: Prentice-Hall International, pp. 233-257.

Evans, John H. (2000): "A sociological account of the growth of principlism", in: Hastings Center Report, September–October, pp. 31-38.

Flynn, Patricia (1991): Moral ordering and the social construction of bioethics. Unpublished doctoral thesis, University of California, San Francisco.

Fost, Norman/Cranford, Ronald E. (1985): "Hospital ethics committees. Administrative aspects", in: Journal of the American Medical Association 253(18), pp. 2687-2692.

Fox, Renee C. (1996): "More than bioethics", in: Hastings Center Report, November-December, pp. 5-7.

— (1990): The evolution of American bioethics: a sociological perspective, in: Weisz, George (eds): Social science perspectives on medical ethics, The Netherlands: Kluwer Academic Publishers, pp. 201-217.

— (1989): The Sociology of Medicine. A participant observer's view, New Jersey: Prentice-Hall International.

Fox, Renee C./Swazey, Judith P. (1984): "Medical morality is not bioethics. Medical ethics in China and the United States", in: Perspectives in Biology and Medicine 27, pp. 337-360.

Joint Commission on the Accreditation of Healthcare Organizations (JCAHO), Accreditation manual for hospitals, Oakbrook Terrace III 1992.

Katz-Rothman, Barbara (2001): The book of life, Boston: Beacon Press.

Kohlen, Helen (2009): Conflicts of care. Hospital ethics committees in the USA and in Germany, Frankfurt a.M.: Campus.

McCormick, Richard A. (1984): "Ethics committees: promise or peril?", in: Law, Medicine & Health Care 12(4), pp. 150-155.

Moreno, Jonathan D. (1995): Deciding together. Bioethics and moral consensus, Oxford: Oxford University Press.

Murphy, Patricia (1989): "The role of the nurse on hospital ethics committees", in: Nursing Clinics of North America 24(2), pp. 551-555.

Pellegrino, Edmund D./Thomasma, David C. (1988): For the patient's good. Oxford: Oxford University Press.

President's Commission for the Study of Ethical Problems in Medicine and Biomedical and Behavioural Research (1983): Deciding to forego life-sustaining treatment, Washington D.C.

Rosner, Fred (1985): "Hospital medical ethics committees. A review of their development", in: Journal of the American Medical Association 253(18), pp. 2693-7.

Ross, Judith W. (1986): Handbook for hospital ethics committees. Practical suggestions for ethics committee members to plan, develop, and evaluate their roles and responsibilities, Chicago: American Hospital Publishing.

Rothman, David (2003): Strangers at the bedside: A history of how law and bioethics transformed medical decision-making, New York: Aldine de Gruyter.

Sichel, Betty A. (1992): Ethics of caring and the institutional ethics committee, in: Bequaert Holmes, Helen/Purdy, Laura M. (eds): Feminist perspectives in medical ethics, Indianapolis: Indiana University Press, pp. 113-123.

Stevens, Tina M.L. (2000): Bioethics in America. Origins and cultural politics, Baltimore: John Hopkins University Press.

Teel, Karen (1975): "The physician's dilemma. A doctor's view. What the law should be", in: Baylor Law Review 27, pp. 6-9.

Thomasma, David C. (1994): Toward a new medical ethics. Implications for ethics in nursing, in: Benner, P. (ed): Interpretative phenomenology, embodiment, caring, and ethics in health and illness, Newbury Park CA: Sage Publications, pp. 85-97.

Tulsky, James A./Fox, Ellen (1996): "Evaluating ethics consultation. Framing the questions", in: The Journal of Clinical Ethics 7(2), pp. 109-115.

Veatch, Robert M. (1977): Hospital ethics committees. Is there a role?, in: Hastings Center Report 7, pp. 22-25.

Walker, Margaret Urban (1993): "Keeping moral space open. Images of ethics consulting", in: Hastings Center Report, March–April, pp. 33-44.

Warren, Virginia L. (1992): Feminist directions in medical ethics, in: Bequaert Holmes, Helen/Purdy, Laura M. (eds): Feminist perspectives in medical ethics, Indianapolis: Indiana University Press, pp. 32-45.

Wolpe, Paul R. (1998): The triumph of autonomy in American bioethics. A sociological view, in: DeVries, Raymond/Subedi, Janardan (eds): Bioethics and society. Constructing the ethical enterprise, New Jersey: Prentice-Hall International, pp. 38-57.

A speaking cure for conflicts: problematization, discourse stimulation and the ongoing of scientific 'progress'[1]

SVEA LUISE HERRMANN

Embryonic stem cell research and research cloning belong to the most contested areas of science and technology, areas which provoke great public and political conflict in many countries. In response to these conflicts, actors, including governments and government institutions, civil society organizations, NGOs, and professional scientific organizations, as well as individuals, demand and initiate public discourses and invite wide participation in ethical deliberation on science and its applications. In the area of the biosciences, particularly, we find a remarkable increase in discursive procedures, institutionalized discourses and new participatory modes of governance that include the public. And, we can observe that science issues

---

1 A speaking cure for conflicts: problematization, discourse stimulation and the ongoing of scientific 'progress', first published in Critical Policy Studies, Vol 4, No. 3, 2010, pp. 278-296. copyright © Institute of Local Government Studies, University of Birmingham reprinted by permission of (Taylor & Francis Ltd, http://www.tandf.co.uk/journals) on behalf of Institute of Local Government Studies, University of Birmingham. I thank the Heinrich Böll-Stiftung for funding part of this research, and the anonymous reviewers of CPS for their valuable comments and Helen Hancock for editing this article.

are increasingly interpreted as 'ethical' issues: struggles in this field are interpreted as 'ethical' conflicts; and new participatory modes, institutions and discursive processes dealing with these issues are defined as 'ethical' debates. The establishment and initiation of these procedures and 'ethical' discourses draw on an assumption that public, 'ethical' debate on science can help to find measures for societal control of scientific endeavor or 'progress'. On the one hand, they are understood as ways of finding measures to limit the potentially damaging effects of new technologies and as ways to alleviate conflicts surrounding techno-scientific developments; on the other, they are interpreted as ways to defy paternalistic and expert-dominated science policy, and too much state power and a lack of transparency and democracy in science policy-making. Seen in this light, public ethical discourses appear to challenge societal power configurations, and to propose societal measures of control for scientific developments.

However, looking at the outcome of public policy discourses on embryonic stem cell research in Great Britain and Germany, we see that (public) 'ethics' discourses do not necessarily lead to control and limitations, but rather to the liberalization of science and its applications. Thus, while we can observe a shift towards more discourse, participation, transparency, and openness in the formulation of science policy, and an increase in references to 'ethics', this does not lead to more societal control of scientific development. The analogous situation in the two countries under study is particularly interesting as, in international comparisons of attitudes to science, they are usually considered to offer opposing examples: Germany is considered an example of 'restrictiveness'; while Great Britain stands for a liberal and very permissive approach to scientific endeavor. Looking at the two cases from the inside, however, a different picture appears and we observe a tendency to liberalization in both countries.[2] On the one hand, this reflects the processes through which the issue came to be *problematized* as an *'ethical'* one concerning the status of the embryo. On the other, it is related to the constant *stimulation* and widening of public 'ethical' debate. In this paper, I suggest that these developments were grounded in, and supported, an im-

---

2   Indeed, it seems that most countries in the world which have regulation of biosciences and biotechnologies in place are moving towards more liberal approaches. Thus, the case studies on Great Britain and Germany illustrate a more widespread trend. I thank the anonymous CPS reviewer for this hint.

perative of scientific progress, and thus complied with the deregulation of scientific endeavor.

For this study, I conducted an interpretive policy discourse analysis focussing on the question of how actors had defined, presented, and interpreted the issue of embryonic stem cell research and research cloning. I analysed documents, reports, and statements produced by actors such as the state and adjacent bodies, stakeholder groups and NGOs, as well as newspaper articles, parliamentary debates and (grey) literature. Additionally, I conducted interviews with concerned actors, such as members of ethics councils, NGOs, and MPs, and I reviewed replies to a public consultation held in Great Britain in 1998.

THE PROBLEMATIZATION OF NEW RESEARCH IN GERMANY AND GREAT BRITAIN

The debates in Great Britain and Germany on embryonic stem cell research and research cloning began in the mid-1990s and ended at the beginning of the new millennium with more permissive regulation of research practice:[3] In 2001, Great Britain permitted research cloning; and in 2002, Germany allowed the import of, and research on, human embryonic stem cells. Despite great differences between the two countries, both debates led in the same direction: that is towards more liberal regulation of techno-scientific development. Differences most obviously concerned the legal side of the issue: the two countries were located at the opposite ends of a scale, with German law, in the form of the Embryo Protection Act (EschG),[4] being very restrictive, and prohibiting embryo research altogether, and British law, in the form of the Human Fertilisation and Embryology Act (HFE Act), being very permissive, while having a comprehensive regulatory framework. At the societal level, the most obvious and important difference concerned the existence and strength, or otherwise, of opposition to, and

---

3   Clearly, the identification of 'the beginning' or 'end' of policy debates is a rather superficial endeavour as 'new' debates always build on 'older' ones as well as providing grounds for yet more debate.
4   Act for the Protection of Embryos (The Embryo Protection Act) of 13th December 1990 (*Embryonenschutzgesetz*).

critiques of, techno-scientific developments: Germany had a strong techno-skeptical community that had emerged in the 1980s and that not only campaigned against certain scientific developments and the lowering of embryo protection, but was also very critical of bioethics discourses. Great Britain, on the other hand, did not have this type of techno-skepticism in the area of human genetics or embryo research. Although in Britain there exists quite a strong alliance against agricultural genetics, this is not the case for human genetics or embryo experimentation (Gaskell et al. 2003). Consequently, debates surrounding the widening of embryo research regulation were much less conflict-ridden than were the German debates on whether research on embryonic stem cells should be permitted. Notwithstanding this difference, policy debates on new research practices in both countries overlapped to a remarkable degree with regard to how the new scientific practices were framed, as well as with regard to the solutions offered. In both countries, the issues at stake were increasingly problematized as *'ethical'* issues concerning *the status of the embryo*; and in both countries more public discourse was demanded and stimulated as a solution to the problem.

PROBLEMATIZATION IN TERMS OF ETHICS

Although today it seems almost 'natural' that biomedical or bioscientific issues should be considered 'ethical' issues, the integration of 'ethics' or 'ethical' questions into policymaking is itself a development calling for attention: Most, if not all, socio-political issues imply normative claims or values, without necessarily being framed as 'ethical'. The great nuclear power conflicts, or conflicts surrounding genetically modified organisms (GMO), were marked by conflicts of value; but these were framed as issues of 'risk' rather than of 'ethics' (Beck 1992). In the nuclear power debates of the 1980s in particular, risk- and not ethics-discourse was the medium in which conflicts were carried out. The notion of 'ethics' had been introduced into policy debates and policymaking in the context of new developments in human genetic technology or in-vitro fertilization (IVF) at the beginning of the 1980s (Braun et al. 2010).

Thus it makes more sense to understand 'ethics' as a 'frame' in Rein and Schön's (1993) sense. Framing, as they define it, is a "way of selecting, organizing, interpreting, and making sense of a complex reality to provide guideposts for knowing, analysing, persuading, and acting" (Rein and Schön 1993: 146). It affects ways of understanding a (problematic) situation and directs attention and channels policy discourse and policy-making in a particular direction (cf. also Fischer 2003; Hajer and Wagenaar 2003; Laws and Rein 2003).

From this point of view, the problematization (Bacchi 1999) of a particular issue/situation is not simply a question of identifying it as problematic but involves the creative act of problem construction. It provides the grounds for, and directs efforts to deal with and solve, certain situations defined as problematic (cf. Hajer and Wagenaar 2003, 13). Problematization, and not just the devising of solutions, are thus both areas of fierce struggle (cf. Fraser 1989a, 1989b). Problematization is a conflict-ridden, discursive process in which various actors struggle over the meaning and definition of 'the problem' and in which 'the problem' is constantly reframed.

Public policy debates on embryonic stem cell research and research cloning in Great Britain and Germany between the mid-1990s and 2002 are examples of struggles over problematization, although to different degrees. Beginning in 1997 with the announcement of the birth of Dolly, the cloned sheep, in The Observer (McKie 1997), a policy debate took place in Great Britain that ended in 2001 with the introduction of the Human Fertilisation and Embryology (Research Purposes) Regulations. Since then, research cloning has been allowed in the UK. In Germany too there were debates in the mid-1990s, initiated by medical professionals, in which permission was demanded to perform pre-implantation genetic diagnosis; and a few years later these were reignited by scientific professionals demanding permission to import human embryonic stem cells for research purposes. The German debate resulted in the implementation of a new Stem Cell Act in 2002 that allowed imports of, and research on, embryonic stem cells on a case-by-case basis. In both countries, debates ended with the liberalization of scientific research practice. Looking more closely at public policy discourses in Great Britain and Germany (cf. Herrmann 2009) we see that the problematizations of human embryonic stem cell research or research cloning were by no means straightforward or unanimous; indeed, the problematizations themselves were the subject of heated disagreements throughout the debates. The new scientific developments turned out to be what Frank Fischer had called "wicked problems", i.e. problems "in which we not only don't know the solution but are not even sure what the problem is" (Fischer 2000:

128). Despite many differences, what public debates on reprogenetics in both countries had in common (although to different degrees) was a plurality of problematizations in the beginning, with the transformation of the dominant problematizations, as well as the narrowing down of the scope of problematizations towards a focus on the moral status of the embryo at the end.

The British debate began after the announcement of the birth of Dolly, the cloned sheep. Although media attention lessened after a while, until the end of 2000 the topic of human cloning recurred intermittently in the context of different, more-or-less-related issues and events.[5] Government actors and high-ranking policy bodies, such as the Science and Technology Committee (STC) of the UK Parliament, the Human Fertilisation and Embryology Authority (HFEA), or the Government itself, were involved in the debates from the beginning. These actors problematized issues such as *the potential of public concerns about science to block scientific development* (e.g. STC 1997a); *an overemphasis on the risks of new technologies in public debates* (e.g. Campbell and Deech 1998) or *a conflict between the status of the embryo and the societal benefits of science* (e.g. DoH 2000a). Others problematized *science out of control* (Joseph Rotblat as quoted in Arlidge 1997) or *an expert-bias in science policy* (Johnson 1997) and demanded that "scientists must take responsibility for their work" (cf. Evening Standard 1997). Later in the debates, the issues of *serious diseases* and *the status of the embryo* (DoH 2000a) were most prominent.

The German struggle was much more adversarial in character than the one in Great Britain. This was due to the existence of a strong techno-skeptical community which interpreted the problem quite distinctly from the techno-optimists.[6] The debate in Germany on the Embryo Protection Act started when professional techno-optimist actors wanted to perform hitherto prohibited practices, i.e. pre-implantation genetic diagnosis (PGD), and a few years later embryonic stem cell research. They problematized *legal restrictions on science as research impediments* (e.g. DFG 1996), or *that scientific innovation might face public reservations* (Caesar 1999). Techno-skeptical actors referred to *the negative social consequences of new re-*

---

5   For an analysis of newspaper coverage cf. Wilkie and Graham (2001) and Kitzinger et al. (2005).
6   On the German techno-skeptical community cf. also Braun (2000).

search fields (ReproKult 2002d), or to the possibility of a *slippery slope towards even more dubious research* (Kollek 1999). Feminist techno-skeptics problematized *the illegitimate instrumentalization of women's needs in order to support scientific research* (Berg et al. 2001). Later, *a conflict between human dignity and the economic potential of embryonic stem cell research* (e.g. Schröder 2000) or *a conflict between the status of the embryo versus the freedom of research* (e.g. Markl 2001) were at the centre of debate. Thus, given the plurality of problematizations, despite differences in scope in both countries, it makes more sense to speak of struggles about problematizations rather than merely of conflicts about solutions. Nevertheless, despite a variety of problematizations in both countries in the beginning, their scope and number were increasingly narrowed down towards the end. Struggles about problematizations in both countries ended with the problematization of *the moral status of the embryo and a plurality of views towards this status*. This 'problem' then appeared as *the* problem.

Problematization and discourse stimulation

The narrowing down of the scope of problematizations towards a focus on the status of the embryo in policy debates in Great Britain and Germany was accompanied by a constant demand for, and an increase in, public (ethical) debate. All actors, including supporters and opponents of the new research, agreed that public debate was critical to deal with 'the problem'. In both countries, we can observe the proliferation of public debates, consultations and conferences, and the establishment of councils or committees to deal with the issue. On the one hand, these had the task of deliberating on 'ethical' questions of biomedical developments; on the other, they were expected to stimulate and foster public debate and encourage the participation of the public. Public debate and participation were seen as appropriate ways to overcome conflicts and to find widely acceptable ways of governing scientific developments.

Authors such as Alan Irwin (2006) or Carr and Levidow (1997) have hinted at the ambivalences and limitations of the new participatory modes in the government of scientific developments. They have particularly pointed to the fact that today public discourse, participation, transparency or public (ethical) deliberation are central elements in science policy,[7] supported by governments and medical and scientific professionals. Public (ethical) discourses are not merely or necessarily the result of emancipative demands by social movements or underrepresented and powerless social actors. Indeed, today, powerful social actors who command social as well as material resources and who are supportive of scientific developments, including governments, policymakers and scientific and medical professionals, themselves refer to social values advocate openness, transparency and integration (cf. Irwin and Michael 2003: 52; Irwin 2006), and demand more public debate. As Alan Irwin (2006) has emphasized, the increasing establishment of deliberation processes and institutions and the proliferation of public (ethical) debate cannot be taken simply as a shift from "technocracy to democracy". The proliferation of public discourses is not necessarily a means of emancipation from power. On the contrary, the stimulation of public discourse can serve the stabilization of power configurations rather than challenging them (cf. also Braun et al. 2010).

Germany

The German debate on PGD and embryonic stem cell research appeared against the background of a strong anti-bioethics/-biomedicine discourse that had turned against unrestricted biomedical 'progress' and utilitarian bioethics (cf. Braun and Herrmann 2000; Herrmann 2009: 135ff). This alliance not only protested against new bioscientific developments but also strongly problematized intransparency, the dominance of experts, and the clandestine manner in which policy decisions on bioscience were taken (e.g. Fuchs 1998; 1999). As a response, they demanded more public debate on the issues at stake under the heading: *What concerns everybody must be decided by everyone*.[8] The alliance believed that more discourse would allow techno-skeptical views to enter the arena of decision-making and strengthen opposition to new biomedical practices, which in their view en-

---

7   On the increase in discursive and participatory procedures at the level of public policy cf. Fairclough (1992); Carr and Levidow (1997); Braun/Herrmann (2000); Hajer and Wagenaar (2003) and Irwin (2006).
8   Cf. Bürger gegen Bioethik, available from: http://www.fuente.de/bioethik [Accessed 8 February 2007).

dangered human rights and dignity – practices such as embryo research or research on people unable to consent (e.g. Grafenecker Erklärung [1995], 1998; Südwest Presse Ulm 2000). They problematized non-democratic decision-making processes which involved exclusively expert discourses. They thought this could (partly) be resolved by means of more inclusive, more open discourses. The demand for more discourse, however, was not in itself understood to be a solution, but was linked to a demand for the restriction and control of scientific research and its application: techno-skeptics insisted on "strict controls" for biomedical research (Grafenecker Erklärung [1995], 1998): "a general prohibition on research on disabled people. [...] Indeed, this is what we demand" (Südwest Presse Ulm 2000).

In the mid-1990s a 'new' debate on PGD emerged which was later superseded by the issue of embryonic stem cell research.[9] This debate was initiated by techno-optimist actors who promoted the new practices hitherto forbidden by the Embryo Protection Act. Professional scientific and medical organizations such as the German Research Foundation (*Deutsche Forschungsgemeinschaft*, DFG) (DFG 1996), the Society for Human Genetics (*Deutsche Gesellschaft für Humangenetik*, GfH) (GfH 1995) or the Federal Medical Association (*Bundesärtzekammer*, BÄK) (BÄK 1998) and individual medical and scientific professionals (cf. Oehmichen 1999) issued statements in which they problematized the prohibition of PGD and embryonic stem cell research in the EschG as instances of "(over)regulation" of research through law (DFG 1996: 1008). They hinted at the presumed negative effects for "freedom of research" (ibid.) or for the couples involved (Oehmichen 1999; DFG 1999). The DFG demanded that the "legislator should hold back" in the area of science and research in favor of "self-government by science", in order to secure "freedom of research" in Germany (DFG 1996: 1011) . While state regulation was problematized, professional self-government was presented as a more rational and effective alternative (BÄK 2001). At the same time, these actors emphasized that the opinion-building process on 'ethical' questions was still in its initial stages

---

9   On 7 July 2010 the German Federal Supreme Court of Justice decided that PGD is *'not liable to prosecution'* if applied to detect a serious genetic disorder (Bundesgerichtshof 2010). Thus, PGD is now *de facto* allowed in Germany, despite the fierce conflicts and debates surrounding it.

and suggested that a broad public debate on the issues should take place (DFG 1999: 6).

Many techno-skeptical actors engaged in the debate, problematizing in particular the socio-political consequences of allowing PGD or embryonic stem cell research. They emphasized, for example, the negative consequences for women (Kollek 1999; Graumann 2000; ReproKult 2002c) and disabled people (Tolmein 1998; ReproKult 2002a), and the danger of a slippery slope towards more dubious applications such as germ-line intervention (Tolmein 1998; Kollek 1999). Techno-skeptics disagreed with the proposition that professional self-regulation should play a prominent role. Instead, they defended restrictive state policy and rejected attacks on the EschG as unacceptable professional encroachments (e.g. ReproKult 2002b; 2002c).

Several more-or-less-official bodies dealt with the topic, and quite a few conferences, symposiums (e.g. BMG 2001) and other processes were initiated in order to find ways of handling societal conflicts and dealing with the new technologies and practices. This was accompanied by an extensive discussion in the media.[10] Despite an intense public debate, many, if not most, commentators and actors demanded more, wider and more open public discourse on the issues. The upsurge in discourse was accompanied by a serious change at its semantic level. Around this time, we can observe a significant narrowing down of issues, and problematizations entering the debates. Before 2000, the debate encompassed a wide range of issues, such as the status and problems of children selected or designed via reprogenetic techniques; the commercialization of the female body as a resource for 'harvesting' egg cells or embryos (Graumann 2002a); the increase in discrimination against, and the decrease of solidarity with, disabled people (Tolmein 1998; ReproKult 2002a); health issues (GfH 1995; Caesar 1999), and the needs and wishes of the couples concerned (GfH 1995) and of science (DFG 1996), and more. At the beginning of the new Millennium, debates in newspapers as well as actors' statements focused much more narrowly on the 'status of the embryo' (cf. also Graumann 2002b). In particu-

---

10 Newspapers articles on bioscience issues increased tenfold in 2000/2001 as compared with the years 1995 to 1999 inclusive (Graumann 2002b: 13). The weekly newspaper *Die Zeit* played a considerable part in the debate. The online version has a big archive of articles at http://www.zeit.de/.

lar, what was no longer problematized was the question of whether or not scientific research should proceed. This narrowing down was induced inter alia by an intervention by Chancellor Gerhard Schröder in December 2000, two days after the British decision to allow research cloning. Schröder declared that it was time to do away with "ideological blinkers" and "general prohibitions" in science policy, and not to lose sight of the international market (Schröder 2000). In a newspaper interview Schröder stated that economic goals were indeed 'ethical goals' (Frankfurter Allgemeine Zeitung 2001). He considered scientific 'progress' to be not only inevitable but necessary for the well-being of a liberal and democratic society. "Progress", he argued, should not be ruled out by legal "constraints" (Schröder 2000). General restrictions for scientific research, from his point of view, would contradict the liberal and economic interests of the nation. He called for a "truly public debate" (*Frankfurter Allgemeine Zeitung* 2001) as, in his view: "It is the task of a democratic society to impede an oligarchy of knowledge—not by prohibition but by educating the general public" (Schröder 2000).

A second intervention came from the designated Minister of Cultural Affairs, Julian Nida-Rümelin, who concentrated on the question of the 'human dignity of the embryo':

The respect for human dignity is appropriate, given the fact that the dignity of a human being can be violated, that his/her self-esteem can be removed. Therefore, the criterion for human dignity cannot be extended to embryos. The self-esteem of human embryos cannot be violated. (Nida-Rümelin 2001)

The article provoked an outcry amongst the German public: actors were outraged that an incumbent minister should publicly annul the principle of human dignity—not only for embryos but, most importantly, for all human beings unequipped with self-esteem (Spaemann 2001: 47). Nida-Rümelin's and Schröder's interventions not only called for and stimulated discourse but, at the same time, promoted and strengthened a framing of embryo research as an issue concerning *the status of the embryo*. They introduced a problematization that centered on questions of whether or not the embryo can be said to possess human dignity, and whether or not it has the right to life. At the same time, and most explicitly in Schröder's interventions, scientific developments were declared to be inevitable and necessary for societal wellbeing. Framing the issue in this way meant that actors on both sides had to articulate their arguments in terms of the status of the embryo. Particularly, feminist techno-skeptics felt compelled, as a matter of strategy, to get involved in the debates (Herrmann and Kurmann 2002; Repro-Kult 2002d). While feminists rejected "concentrating on 'the protection of life' in the public debate" (ReproKult 2002d: 120), getting involved in legal debates on the embryo was nevertheless seen as necessary for strategic reasons.[11]

Although the discourse exploded in 2000, calls for more, more rational and more public, as well as more institutionalized, debates nevertheless increased. Two new 'ethics' boards were set up. The establishment of the parliamentary Enquête-Commission on the Law and Ethics of Modern Medicine (EK REM) had been demanded by the anti-bioethics alliance as a response to what they believed to be a lack of democratic legitimacy. The parliamentary commission was meant to counter a lack of public discourse on biomedicine policy. The National Ethics Council (NEC), established by Chancellor Schröder, was the result of calls for a "new discourse" from within the Government. This new discourse was supposed to be "more rational" and "less disordered and emotional" (Catenhusen 2001) than the existing one. As health minister Ulla Schmidt said, a national ethics council should be "the place for responsible discussion at the executive level" (Schmidt 2001) and the new discourse should explicitly *replace* a decision: "If we don't know as a society where to set the ethical and cultural boundaries, new prohibitions don't make any sense" (Schmidt quoted in *Frankfurter Rundschau* 2001). Despite their different origins, both boards were the result of calls for more or new debates. Their task was to organize and structure public debate (Deutscher Bundestag 2001; German National Ethics Council 2001) in order to ease the strong conflicts on the issue within the German public.

However, which conflict? As has been mentioned above, the scope and number of problematizations current amongst the German public had seri-

---

11 The focus on the embryo brought back "the abortion question", a link that feminists have always rejected. Techno-skeptical feminists argued that pregnancy was a special situation that could not be compared, including in legal terms, with any other situation, because the embryo only existed in and by means of the pregnant woman (cf. Mildenberger 2002; Braun 2003).

ously decreased over the years, leading to a focus on the embryo. The subject of ethical deliberation, both commissions stressed, was *the status of the embryo*. More precisely, conflicts within the public, both agreed, were the result of *a plurality of ethical views towards the status of the embryo* (German National Ethics Council 2001: 10f; Deutscher Bundestag 2001: 30, 51). At the same time, however, different 'ethical' views on this status were interpreted as irreconcilable. As the EK REM stated: "it is impossible to foresee when in the future dissent over the moral status of the human embryo in vitro will be eliminated" (Deuscher Bundestag 2001: 43).

Scientific 'progress' on the other hand was interpreted as given and unquestionable. Indeed, the two boards' reports were based on the assumption that the need for 'ethical' evaluation of stem cell research and imports *arose* from developments and prospects in science and technology and their potential applications, and not vice versa.[12] Besides current developments, "the expected *future developments*" in the new research (Deutscher Bundestag 2001: 16, emphasis added) and the "hoped for" results of experiments that might "one day" be arrived at (German National Ethics Council 2001: 9) formed the background to the 'ethical' evaluation in both commissions. The NEC said its task was to "assess *the possible consequences of scientific and technological innovations,*[…] and [to] reflect on the significance of *the opportunities created by science and technology*" (German National Ethics Council 2001: 10, emphasis added). Thus, that science and technology *will* proceed, and that there *will* be "hoped for" "future developments" or "opportunities", was the prerequisite for ethical deliberation and was itself beyond contestation.

Despite the assumption of the irreconcilability of the 'ethical' conflict, or because of it, both commissions considered a certain solution to be appropriate. This was, however, not a substantial but a practical solution: *public debate*. As the chair of the NEC stated, it was not the responsibility of the council to provide "definite answers" but the council was instead "an authority for stimulating discussion" (personal Interview with S. Simitis, 27 Oct 2005 in Berlin). The NEC saw its main task as facilitating understanding of the new research and triggering public debate because:

---

12 Parliament had emphasised that, as a *result* of 'developments in the field of genetics', there was a need for 'ethical evaluation' of embryonic stem cell research (BT DR 14/6551).

Everyone must be able to form an impression of the prospects and risks of the new technologies, as a basis for arriving at his or her *own judgment* on the associated ethical issues." (German National Ethics Council 2001: 7, emphasis added)

The public was invited to participate in ethical debate, not to arrive at a common solution, but so that each person could form *their own* perspective on the issues. In fact, the possibility (at least in the foreseeable future) of arriving at a mutual solution to the 'ethical' question of the status of the embryo was excluded. Precisely the fact that the conflict was framed as an *ethical* issue, that 'ethical' views were interpreted as irreconcilable, and that finding a common answer was declared impossible, underpinned calls for more public debate.

In the parliamentary debates at the end of January 2002, MPs could decide between three motions: one calling for a total ban on embryonic stem cell research (BT DR 14/8101); one calling for its approval (BT DR 14/8103); and a third motion – the one parliament voted for – which included a general prohibition on the creation and import of, and research on, human embryonic stem cells, but at the same time allowed certain regulated exceptions (BT DR 14/8102).[13] While this 'no-but' decision was certainly a compromise circumventing the two extremes, it was nonetheless a decision for permitting embryonic stem cell research in Germany.

In March 2002 the Stem Cell Act (StZG)[14] was passed allowing imports of embryonic stem cells if certain criteria were met. Most importantly, embryonic stem (ES) cells must have been produced outside Germany before January 2002 (*Stichtagsregelung*). Secondly, a newly established Central Commission for Stem Cell Research (*Zentrale Ethikkommission für Stammzellforschung*, ZES) must have approved the research on a case-by-case basis. This commission is the first 'ethics' body in Germany that actually has the authority to make a decision similar to the British Human Fertilisation and Embryology Authority. The Stem Cell Act determines the 'ethical' framework for decision-making, i.e. the arguments and activities that have to be produced and performed by applicants in order to get approval for a

---

13 This motion resembled the minority vote of the EK REM (Deutscher Bundestag 2001: 57ff).

14 Act Ensuring Protection of Embryos in Connection with the Importation and Utilization of Embryonic Stem Cells (The Stem Cell Act) of 28 June 2002.

proposed piece of research on imported ES cells. In short: Parliament provided the rules and frames for the discourse, and the ZES would administer and control adherence to these rules. Thus, parliament abstained from a clear statement pro or contra embryonic stem cell research, but instead referred decision-making to further ethical deliberation under the auspices a new ethics body. Framing the issue in terms of 'ethics' and referring it to the ZES signalled that 'ethical concerns' were taken seriously and measures of 'control' were to be implemented, while simultaneously ensuring that scientific endeavour could proceed. As the chair of the EK REM has pointedly said: "This is how it should be: today we have as many stem cell research centres in Germany as in Great Britain, and no one takes offence at them, despite the angry discussions we had" (personal Interview with M. von Renesse, 19 Jan 2006 in Bochum). Indeed, the deadline set for ES cell production has since been moved forward. Today German researchers are allowed to import ES cells that were produced before May 2007. Since the implementation of the Act, the ZES has approved 50 research applications (ZES 2009). Thus, while the Embryo Protection Act has not been amended, embryo protection has been liberalized by the fact that the Stem Cell Act now allows embryonic stem cell research in Germany.

Great Britain

The British debate on research cloning was much less controversial than the German one. It appeared against a background of growing general skepticism about the ability of politics to govern science and technology developments. While 'red' biotechnology was a much less controversial issue than the 'green' version, nonetheless some actors presumed that the Government's hesitation to quickly make a law allowing research cloning was due to fears that skepticism towards GMO might spill over into issues of embryo research (Sexton 2000). Public conflicts on GMO and the BSE drama (Forbes 2004) were interpreted as crises in policy-making (Gaskell et al. 2003). The public increasingly thought that "government and industry were doing a bad job [...] over biotechnology" (Gaskell et al. 2003). Both crises brought the issue of 'public trust' and the need for public participation into the focus of UK policy-makers (Irwin and Michael 2003; Grove-White 2006). In this context, public skepticism or critique of scientific developments was redefined, from being seen as deriving from a knowledge deficit that could be dealt with by education to becoming a trust deficit calling for participatory measures involving the public (cf. Irwin 2006). Policymakers detected a "crisis of confidence" (Irwin 2006: 307) in science and science-policy leading to the suggestion that the relationship between science and the public needed to be reorganized. The 'crisis' was to be resolved via openness, transparency and public participation. As Carr and Levidow (1997) stated, it was in the context of public debates over agricultural biotechnology that 'risk' discourses were supplemented with 'ethical' ones. 'Ethics' discourses appeared together with the 'recognition' of public (ethical) concerns and a rise in participatory initiatives (Wynne 2001).

While embryo research was relatively uncontested in Great Britain, the announcement of the cloning of Dolly the sheep caused an outbreak of public debate, especially in the press. Many commentators, including both those who supported the new research (Ian Wilmut quoted in Arlidge 1997) and those who were skeptical about it (e.g. Johnson 1997; Bill Cash quoted in Highfield 1997; David Alton quoted in de Bruxelles 1997), demanded a public debate on the issue.

Also, high-ranking policy bodies were involved in the debates from the beginning. A few weeks after the announcement of Dolly's birth, the Science and Technology Committee (STC) of the UK Parliament held a consultation, interviewing members of the University of Edinburgh's Roslin Institute,[15] the Human Fertilisation and Embryology Authority (HFEA), the Department of Health (DoH), and the Ministry of Agriculture, Fisheries and Food (MAFF) and more.[16] At the core of the STC consultation in 1997 (STC 1997a; 1997b), as well as of statements by witnesses, was apprehension that 'irrational fears' and 'public concerns' about science might "block benign developments" (STC 1997a: ix). 'Public confidence' needed to be

---

15 Dolly had been created at Roslin Institute.
16 Including also: memoranda from the Home Office; the Department of Health; the Institution of Professionals, Managers, and Specialists – Biotechnology and Biological Sciences Research Council Branch, Roslin Institute Section; the British Medical Association; the Office of Science and Technology; the Constitutional and Community Policy Directorate within the Home Office; the Institution of Professionals, Managers, and Specialists; and the Roslin Institute together with PPL Therapeutics.

maintained, because "hand in hand with scientific achievements and their potential application come equally significant issues of appropriate regulation and public confidence", as the Office of Science and Technology stated (OST 1997: 43). Public debate lacked balance, it was argued, and 'strong public reaction', especially that conveyed in newspapers, had overshadowed the discussion of the benefits (STC 1997a: ix). Public mistrust needed a response, in order to enhance "the UK's lead in Europe in the industrial exploitation of biotechnology and for the UK to outpace international competitors" (OST 1997: 44). The "Crusade" for biotechnology needed to recognize "the importance of public confidence", the OST said (ibid.). For these bodies it was quite clear that the 'UK's lead in biotechnology' should remain unchallenged. The 'problem' was that lack of public trust might endanger the achievement of this aim. Nevertheless, witnesses in the consultation made clear that particular applications of human cloning "are issues for society, they are not issues for scientists" (Bulfield quoted in STC 1997b: 26).[17] Thus, as a response to public concerns, they suggested to lead "an informed discussion in a debating format" (ibid.: 25). 'Ethics' or 'ethical debate' seemed a promising way to reassure the public without putting scientific 'progress' at risk: As the STC wrote in its final report:[18]

The experience with genetic engineering technology shows that an explicit moratorium can be productive. On the one hand, it sends a public signal that ethical considerations are important and need to be taken into account, and allows that to happen. On the other, the fact that a moratorium is, by definition, likely to be lifted at some point indicates that further development is anticipated. (STC 1997a: x)

The problematization of public concerns, of unbalanced public debate and of the risk of blocking scientific development led the Government to decline to accept the STC's recommendations. Instead, it said that first of all more public debate was needed in order to "maintain public confidence" (DTI and OST 1997: 6), while the "Government will also strive to *ensure that the debate on the ethical issues keeps pace with advances in these technologies*" (DTI and OST 1997: 7 emphasis added). However, the fact that 'public concerns' remained rather vaguely described and were indeed

---

17 Bulfield was then Director and Chief Executive of the Roslin Institute.
18 Quoting from Nature, Mar 6, 1997, Vol. 386: 1.

highly exaggerated indicates that their problematization was a means of underpinning calls for public debate rather than a response to a critique of, or opposition to, science.[19] Against the background of public conflicts on GMO and BSE that had led to a climate of skepticism towards science policy, exaggerating opposing statements and the problematization of public concerns about cloning were means of underpinning calls for a 'new' public debate—a debate that should be characterized by knowledge, rationality, and expert guidance. They were means of stimulating public debate that 'kept pace with science' rather than challenging it. An early public debate was expected to establish public trust in policy-making and to secure "science's license to practice" (Royal Society 2004: 7; cf. Irwin 2006: 308).

The next step in the debate was a public consultation held by the joint cloning working group (CWG) of the HFEA and the HGAC[20] (1998a) which received around 200 responses from organization and individuals.[21] As Ruth Deech (then chair of the HFEA) and Colin Campbell (then chair of the HGAC) wrote: "it is necessary to clear away the hype surrounding cloning and replace it with informed opinion" (Campbell and Deech 1998: 31). Commentary on the Dolly technique, they went on, had been overshadowed by "fears that this technique might open Pandora's box" and the consultation should help to avoid a "knee-jerk reaction" (ibid.). The CWG report made unquestionably clear that "it is our wish that the wide potential benefits of this technology are maximized, while at the same time concerns are recognized and adequate safeguards are implemented" (HFEA and HGAC 1998b: 1). Underlying the consultation process as a whole was a strong commitment to scientific 'progress' which was beyond problematization and needed to be communicated to the public through their engagement in debate. The consultation, in Alan Irwin's terms, served to set up a "framework for engagement" (Irwin 2006: 316) and was expected to help to 'improve informed debate'. As a result, the CWG identified "the need for more education and informed debate" (HFEA and HGAC 1998b: 20).

---

19 Although there was some criticism of 'human cloning', overall there was much more emphasis in the press on the benefits, rather than the risks involved or the concerns raised (cf. Wilkie and Graham 2001; Kitzinger and Williams 2005).
20 Human Genetic Advisory Commission.
21 The responses have not been published. I have sifted through them in the Department of Health where they are kept.

Again, the Government did not accept the report but stated that further consideration and debate was needed before decisions could be made (DoH 1999). The cloning issue was therefore handed over to another deliberative committee, the Chief Medical Officer's expert advisory group. Under the title Stem Cell Research: Medical Progress with Responsibility, the expert group was to discuss the 'benefits' and 'risks' of the new research, the 'ethical and social implications' and the question of whether or not the HFE Act needed to be amended to include the new research (DoH 2000a, annex A). The focus of the expert consultation was: the technology is here; now what can we do with it?

The most significant contribution of the CMO expert group was to introduce into the debate a new problematization, namely the problematization of *'serious diseases'* such as chronic illnesses or organ failure as a severe social problem (DoH 2000a: 16). Although the so-called possibilities of research cloning had been mentioned before, they had been rather vaguely defined. The CMO report clearly problematized 'serious diseases' as a societal problem in need of a solution. At the same time, it presented research cloning as the appropriate answer, and through this move transformed research cloning into the solution. Nevertheless, although presented as a solution without alternatives to the problem of serious diseases, the expected results of research cloning were depicted in highly speculative ways:

It is *envisaged* that tissues developed from stem cells derived from embryos created by cell nuclear replacement *would* have the advantage of being free from rejection because they *should* be genetically compatible with the person being treated [...]. *If this proves to be the case*, there is a great *potential* benefit to human health. (DoH 2000a: 23 emphasis added)

The speculative nature of the anticipated goals supported the call for more research. More research would, the group suggested, "enable a better assessment to be made of the true potential of the research" (DoH 2000a: 31). Thus both levels of problematization—that of 'serious diseases' and that of 'uncertainty of research'—were presented as requiring the same answer, that is, more research.

Through transforming research cloning into a solution to serious diseases, any other problems with cloning were transformed into ones of a second order—subdivided into technical and ethical problems. Following the interpretation of Carr and Levidow (1997), the former were interpreted as belonging to the domain of objective science and expertise, and the latter to the realm of 'irreconcilable moral beliefs'. In this way, 'ethical' problems, such as concerns or unease, were addressed without having a serious impact on the 'technical' side. Thus any more general questioning of embryo research was excluded. Whether or not embryo research should proceed could not be problematized. What the CMO group presented as *the* moral question was the status of the embryo: while the use of embryos, the group said, "raises important ethical issues for many people" (DoH 2000a: 13), it concluded, however, that it was "not possible to reconcile the opposing views on the moral status of the embryo and on the use of embryos in research" (DoH 2000a: 39). In its conclusion, the group said that "the potential benefits of the research could be weighed against the respect owed to the embryo, given its very early stage of development" (DoH 2000a: 41) and it recommended that research cloning be allowed. This time, the British Government accepted the recommendations in full. It stressed however, that it "respects the view of those people who believe that human embryos should not be used in any research" (DoH 2000b: 4).

Problematization of serious diseases and of irreconcilable moral views about the status of the embryo also formed the background to the parliamentary debates that followed the CMO report (cf. also Herrmann 2003). In particular, framing research cloning as an issue of '*individual* ethical/moral beliefs' was decisive for the form as well as the outcome of the parliamentary debates: MPs agreed that they should 'speak only for themselves' (e.g. David Wilshire, HC Deb, 19 Dec 2000: col. 246) and that they "fully accept the validity of arguments advanced by other hon. Members with different points of view" (Edward Leigh, HC Deb, 19 Dec 2000: col. 258). The new research was framed as a matter of personal moral conviction rather than an issue of "party politics" (Michael Fabricant, HC Deb, 15 Dec 2000: col. 919). This meant the exclusion of claims that a certain conviction was "right" while others were declared to be "wrong". Indeed, any claim of certainty about judgments appeared as a "moral imposition" and "fundamentalism". As the conservative MP Robert Key said, "[i]f we are not careful we become fundamentalists hanging on to a few dogmas that we do not intend to examine and which we will not give up" (HC Deb, 17 Nov 2000: col. 1216). The framing of the new research as an issue of *individual ethical* conviction inherently meant the refusal to make a definite judgment or to arrive at a common political resolution. One MP voting in favor of the new research quoted from a letter she wrote to a community of nuns:

One of the things that I envy in people like the members of your community, who have a faith, is that you have the comfort of having certainty about these questions. I have to try to work out how to balance the different arguments. (Fiona MacTaggert, HC Deb, 19 Dec 2000: col. 247)

The effect of this was that the issue of research cloning was portrayed as a matter of individual moral decision rather than state intervention. As supporters of the new research stated, it was subject to personal moral decisions, a question of the right to choose whether or not to donate eggs or embryos, and whether or not to use therapies derived from embryo research:

Accepting treatment is a personal decision. [...] The whole point about the regulations is that they are permissive [...]. They will not force people to accept the treatment. (Evan Harris, HC Deb, 19 Dec 2000: col. 253)

Within this frame, any claim to restrict scientific endeavor appeared as a 'moral imposition' and, hence, as denying the option of a choice. As Yvette Cooper made clear: "If parliament votes against these regulations, hon. Members will deny couples the *choice to donate* their spare embryos to stem cell research" (HC Deb, 19 Dec 2000: col. 214, emphasis added). Thus, allowing the new research was presented as a pre-requisite for an 'ethical viewpoint' and an individual 'ethical decision'. 'Ethics' meant a personal decision on options provided by scientific research.

In the final decision in the British parliament, problematization of the issue in terms of *individual moral beliefs* lead to the disqualification of general limits to embryonic stem cell research as a 'moral imposition' and as illegitimate intervention in the right to choose. Potential donors to the research, or 'patients' profiting from it, were conceived of as consumers who would decide along the lines of their personal moral convictions. While 'ethics' played an integral part in the parliamentary debates, parliament reclaimed the classic feature of state neutrality towards values, beliefs, and opinions and refrained from state-juridical limitations on research. Limits on research were disqualified as a 'moral impositions' on the grounds of individual autonomy and freedom regarding personal moral beliefs – while scientific 'progress' became the pre-requisite for 'ethical' decisions and could not be challenged or problematized.

Generating the learned participant and 'ethical' consumer

In the policy debate on embryonic stem cell research or research cloning in Great Britain and Germany, we find differences and similarities. Policy debates in both countries differed greatly, particularly with regard to the permissiveness or otherwise of science policy and to the existence and strength of public opposition to the new research. Despite these differences, however, both debates ended in the liberalization of scientific research: Great Britain allowed research cloning; and Germany allowed embryonic stem cell research.

Contrary to the assumption that public ethical debate could help to find measures for controlling scientific developments, 'ethics' did not form a counter-discourse to the commitment to scientific 'progress'. On the contrary, problematization of the issues in terms of ethics strengthened this commitment. Referring (actual or potential) conflicts on science to the area of 'ethics', i.e. framing conflicts as issues of *irreconcilable individual moral beliefs on the status of the embryo*, meant avoidance of the problematization of scientific 'progress'. That science *will* proceed formed the background principle of 'ethical' debate. We are talking about the embryo, not about science! At the same time, the assumption of the irreconcilability of the (individualized) conflict presupposed that a common answer could not and need not be found. This understanding worked in favor of liberal and individualistic market logic. In Great Britain in particular, 'ethics' meant that individuals could choose from a set of options produced by science according to their 'ethical' preferences on such issues as the donation of egg cells or the use of certain therapies—a decision the 'morally neutral' legislator could not take if a 'moral imposition' was to be avoided. Public participation in 'ethical' debates was thus directed at personal decision-making according to the personal moral convictions of the 'ethical' consumer, a process for which scientific 'progress' is a pre-requisite. In Germany, on the other hand, ethical debate was directed at the formation of a personal 'ethical' perspective on the new research. In this regard, it was the task of the National Ethics Council to stimulate discussion and to offer a set of possible 'ethical' positions from which individuals could choose. In Germany as well, parliament refrained from a clear-cut decision on whether or not to allow ES cell research. Instead, it transferred decision-making to a newly established ethics council and provided the discursive rules and standards for deliberation and case-by-case decision-making by the council. Thus both parliaments abstained from direct state intervention in scientific and technological development but instead provided a 'framework for engagement' with new developments—while at the same time securing the way ahead for science.

At the same time, framing conflicts in terms of 'ethics' implied in both countries an invitation to each and everyone to participate in the debate in order to be able to form and articulate their own 'ethical' view or to be able to make an autonomous 'ethical' decision in the face of the options provided by science. Public *ethical* debate provided a space for the *articulation* or *formation* of different perspectives on *the status of the embryo* without, however, providing the possibility of political contestation of scientific 'progress'. In the two countries, public discourse, especially a discourse in terms of 'ethics', was a medium in which an imperative of scientific progress, on the one hand, as well as actual or possible concerns about, or opposition to, scientific endeavor on the other, could coexist. However, the commitment to public engagement, to the integration of (ethical) concerns and critique, to debate, transparency and openness did not exclude a similar commitment to scientific progress.

REFERENCES

Act for the Protection of Embryos (The Embryo Protection Act) of 13th December 1990. Federal Lay Gazette, Part I, No 69, issued in Bonn, 19th December 1990, page 2746. Available from: http://www.bmj.bund.de/files/fe5fef9d2041e75ec37796d8e517288e/1147/ESchG%20englisch.pdf [Accessed 7 June 2010].

Act Ensuring Protection of Embryos in Connection with the Importation and Utilization of Embryonic Stem Cells (The Stem Cell Act) of 28 June 2002 (unofficial translation). Available from: http://www.bmj.bund.de/files/-/1146/Stammzellgesetz%20englisch.pdf [Accessed 2 August 2010].

Arlidge, J., 1997. Scientist 'able to create human clone'. The Guardian, 26 February 1997.
Bacchi, C. L., 1999. Women, policy and politics. The construction of policy problems. London: Sage.
Beck, U., 1992. Risk society: towards a new modernity. London: Sage.
Berg, G., Graumann, S., and Schneider, I., 2001. Fortschrittsgläubiger Rückfall in alte Fronten. Freitag, 2001(3).
BMG, 2001. Bundesministerium der Gesundheit. Fortpflanzungsmedizin in Deutschland. Wissenschaftliches Symposium des Bundesministeriums für Gesundheit in Zusammenarbeit mit dem Robert Koch-Institut, 24.-26. Mai 2000. Berlin: Nomos Verlag.
Braun, K., 2000. Menschenwürde und Biomedizin. Zum Philosophischen Diskurs der Bioethik. Frankfurt a.M.: Campus.
Braun, K., 2003. Embryonen im sozialen Kontext? Die Rolle von geschlechtersensitiven Argumenten und von Frauen als Akteurinnen in der Biomedizindebatte in Deutschland. In Österreichische Zeitschrift für Politikwissenschaft, 32 (2003/2), 137-148.
Braun, K., and Herrmann, S. L., 2000. If discourse is the solution - what is the problem? Paper presented at the ECPR Joint Session of Workshops, Workshop 9: "Policy, Discourse & Institutional Reform", Grenoble, France, 6-11 April 2000 [online]. Available from: http://www.essex.ac.uk/ECPR/events/jointsessions/paperarchive/grenoble/ws9/braun.pdf [Accessed 20 January 2002].
Braun, K., Herrmann, S. L., Moore, A. and Könninger, S., 2010 (forthcoming). Science governance and the politics of proper talk: governmental bioethics as a new technology of reflexive government. In Economy and Society, Vol 3, No. 4, 511-533, (first pulished online, 24 November 2010, as doi:10.1080/03085147.2010.510682).
Bundesärztekammer (BÄK), 1998. Richtlinien zur Durchführung der assistierten Reproduktion. In Deutsches Ärzteblatt, 95(49), 3166-3171.
Bundesärztekammer (BÄK), 2001. Diskussionsentwurf zu einer Richtlinie zur Präimplantationsdiagnostik. In Graumann, S. ed. Die Genkontroverse. Grundpositionen. Freiburg: Herder Spektrum. 157-168.
Caesar, P., 1999. Präimplantationsdiagnostik. Thesen zu den medizinischen, rechtlichen und ethischen Problemstellungen. Bericht der Bioethik-Kommission des Landes Rheinland-Pfalz vom 20. Juni 1999. Alzey: Ministerium der Justiz Rheinland-Pfalz.

Campbell, C., and Deech, R., 1998. Consulting on cloning. In SPA, (Spring), 31-33.
Carr, S., and Levidow, L., 1997. How biotechnology regulation sets a risk/ethics boundary. In Agriculture and human values, 14 (1), 29-43.
Catenhusen, W.-M., 2001. Interview am Morgen. Zum Streit um die neue Gen-Politik. Radio-Interview, Deutschlandfunk. Jan 19.
de Bruxelle, S., 1997. Scientists 'close to recreating the dead'. The Times, 27 February.
Department of Health (DoH), 1999. Government response to the report by the human fertilisation and embryology authority and the human genetics advisory commission on cloning issues in reproduction, science and medicine. London: The Stationery Office.
Department of Health (DoH), 2000a. Stem cell research: medical progress with responsibility. A report form the chief medical officer's expert group reviewing the potential of developments in stem cell research and cell nuclear replacement to benefit human health. London: The Stationery Office.
Department of Health (DoH), 2000b. Government response to the recommendations made in the chief medical officer's expert group report 'stem cell research: medical progress with responsibility'. London: The Stationery Office.
Department of Trade and Industry and Office of Science and Technology (DTI and OST), 1997. The cloning of animals from adult cells— government response to the fifth report of the House of Commons' select committee on science and technology, 1996-97 session. London: The Stationery Office.
Deutsche Forschungsgemeinschaft (DFG), 1996. Forschungsfreiheit - ein Plädoyer der Deutschen Forschungsgemeinschaft für bessere Rahmenbedingungen der Forschung in Deutschland. In Der Frauenarzt, 37(7), 1007-1023.
Deutsche Forschungsgemeinschaft (DFG), 1999. Stellungnahme der Deutschen Forschungsgemeinschaft zum Problemkreis 'Humane embryonale Stammzellen'. In Graumann, S., ed. 2001. Die Genkontroverse. Freiburg: Herder. 107-114.
Deutscher Bundestag, 2001. Zweiter Zwischenbericht der Enquête-Kommission Recht und Ethik der modernen Medizin. Teilbericht Stammzellforschung, BT DR 14/7546. Berlin: Deutscher Bundestag.

Evening Standard, 1997. The folly of Dolly. Nobel Peace Prize Winner Professor Joseph Rotblat talking to Suzie Mackenzie. Evening Standard, 28 February.

Fairclough, N., 1992. Discourse and social change. Cambridge: Polity Press.

Fischer, F., 2000. Citizens, experts, and the environment. Durham and London: Duke University Press.

Fischer, F., 2003. Reframing public policy. Discourse politics and deliberative practice. Oxford: University Press.

Forbes, I., 2004. Making a crisis out of a drama: the political analysis of BSE-policy making in the UK. In Political studies, 52 (2), 342-357.

Frankfurter Allgemeine Zeitung, 2001. Die Notwendigkeit der Abwägung stellt sich immer wieder neu. Interview des Bundeskanzlers zur Bioethik. Frankfurter Allgemeine Zeitung, 3 May.

Frankfurter Rundschau, 2001. Regierung legt Gesetze zum Menschen-Klonen auf Eis. Frankfurter Rundschau, 5 February.

Fraser, N., 1989a. Struggle over needs: outline of a socialist-feminist critical theory of the late capitalist political culture. In Fraser, N., Unruly practices. Power, discourse and gender in contemporary social theory. Minneapolis: University of Minnesota Press, 161-190.

Fraser, N., 1989b. Women, welfare and the politics of need interpretation. In Fraser, N., Unruly practices. Power, discourse, and gender in contemporary social theory. Minneapolis: University of Minnesota Press, 144-160.

Fuchs, U. (1999). Die Ethik der Bio-Macht. Bioethik oder: Tabubrüche hinter verschlossenen Türen. In Emmrich, M., ed. Im Zeitalter der Bio-Macht. 25 Jahre Gentechnik - eine kritische Bilanz. Frankfurt a.M.: Mabuse-Verlag, 261-273.

Fuchs, U., 1998. Experten entscheiden selbst. Unter sich. Und über uns. Die Bio-Ethik-Konvention geht alle an. In Wunder, M. and Neuer-Miebach, T., eds. Bio-Ethik und die Zukunft der Medizin. Bonn: Psychiatrie-Verlag, 130-138

Gaskell, G., Bauer, M. W., Jackson, J., Howard, S., and Lindsey, N., 2003. Ambivalent GM nation? Public attitudes to bin the UK 1991-2002. 'Life sciences in European society' report. London: London School of Economics and Political Sciences.

German National Ethics Council, 2001. The import of human embryonic stem cells. Opinion. Berlin: Nationaler Ethikrat Deutschland.
Gesellschaft für Humangenetik (GfH), 1995. Stellungnahme zur Präimplantationsdiagnostik. In Medizinische Genetik, 7, 420.
Grafenecker Erklärung [1995], 1998. Granfenecker Erklärung zur Bio-Ethik. In Wunder M. and Neuer-Miebach, T., eds. Bio-Ethik und die Zukunft der Medizin. Bonn: Psychiatrie-Verlag, 182-195.
Graumann, S., 2000. Gen-Check vor der Schwangerschaft. Gen-ethischer Informationsdienst GID, 139, 13-16.
Graumann, S., 2002a. Liberation or disempowerment of women—the social consequences of reproductive medicine and genetic diagnosis from the standpoint of women's policy. In ReproKult eds. Reproductive medicine and genetic engineering. Women between self-determination and societal standardisation. Bonn: Bundeszentrale für gesundheitliche Aufklärung, 111-115.
Graumann, S., 2002b. Situation der Medienberichterstattung zu aktuellen Entwicklungen in der Biomedizin und ihren ethischen Fragen [online]. Bioethik-Diskurs. Available from: http://www.bioethik-diskurs.de/documents/wissensdatenbank/gutachten/Berichterstattung.html/view [Accessed 2 August 2010].
Grove-White, R., 2006. Britain's GM crop controversies: the AEBC and the negotiation of 'uncertainty'. In Community genet, 9(3), 170-177.
Hajer, M., and Wagenaar, H., 2003. Introduction. In Hajer, M. and Wagenaar, H., eds. Deliberative policy analysis. Understanding governance in the network society. Cambridge: University Press, 1-30.
Herrmann, S. L. and Kurmann, M., 2002. Foreword. In ReproKult eds. Reproductive medicine and genetic engineering. Women between self-determination and societal standardisation. Bonn: Bundeszentrale für gesundheitliche Aufklärung, 6.
Herrmann, S. L., 2003. Deregulation via regulation. On the moralisation and maturalisation of embryonic stem cell research in the British parliamentary debates of 2000/2001. In Österreichische Zeitschrift für Politikwissenschaft, 32(2003/2), 149-161. Available from: http://www.oezp.at/pdfs/2003-2-03.pdf [Accessed 7 June 2010].
Herrmann, S. L., 2009. Policy debates on reprogenetics. The problematization of new research in Great Britain and Germany. Frankfurt a.M.: Campus.

Highfield, J., 1997. Santer raises concerns over human cloning. Daily Telegraph, 28 February.

Human Fertilisation and Embryology Act 1990. Available from: http://www.opsi.gov.uk/acts/acts1990/Ukpga_19900037_en_1.htm [Accessed 15 January 2010].

Human Fertilisation and Embryology Authority and Human Genetics Advisory Commission (HFEA and HGAC), 1998a. Cloning issues in reproduction, science and medicine—a consultation paper. London: Department of Health.

Human Fertilisation and Embryology Authority and Human Genetics Advisory Commission (HFEA and HGAC), 1998b. Cloning issues in Reproduction, science and medicine - report. London: Department of Health.

Human Fertilisation and Embryology (Research Purposes) Regulations 2001. Available from: http://www.opsi.gov.uk/si/si2001/uksi_20010188_en.pdf [Accessed 7 June 2010].

Irwin, A., 2006. The politics of talk. Coming to terms with the 'new' scientific governance. In Social studies of science, 36 (2), 299-320.

Irwin, A. and Michael, M., 2003. Science, social theory and public knowledge. Maidenhead, Phil.: Open University Press.

Johnson, P., 1997. Age of man-made monsters? Daily Mail, 24 February, Commentary.

Kitzinger, J. and Williams, C., 2005. Forecasting science futures: legitimising hope and calming fears in the embryo stem cell debate. In Social science and medicine, 61 (3), 731-740.

Kollek, R., 1999. Wegen der ethischen Brisanz nicht akzeptabel. Gen-ethischer Informationsdienst GID, 131, 14-16.

Laws, D. and Rein, M., 2003. Reframing Practice. In Hajer, M. and Wagenaar, H., eds. Deliberative policy analysis. Understanding governance in the network society. Cambridge: University Press, 172-206.

Markl, H., 2001. Freiheit, Verantwortung, Menschenwürde, Warum Lebenswissenschaften mehr sind als Biologie. In Geyer, C., ed. Biopolitik. Die Positionen. Frankfurt a.M.: Suhrkamp Verlag, 177-193.

McKie, R., 1997. Scientists clone adult sheep. The Observer, 23 February.

Mildenberger, E. H., 2002. Why unwanted pregnancies, embryo selection and embryo research must generally be treated differently. In Repro-Kult, eds. Reproductive medicine and genetic engineering. Women between self-determination and societal standardisation. Bonn: Bundeszentrale für gesundheitliche Aufklärung, 115-119.

Nida-Rümelin, J., 2001. Wo die Menschenwürde beginnt. Das Klonen von Embryonen: ein Heilsweg oder der Anfang eines gespenstischen Menschenbilds? Auch Deutschland kann einer neuen bio-ethischen Debatte nicht mehr ausweichen. Der Tagesspiegel, 3 January.

Oehmichen, M., 1999. Präimplantationsdiagnostik: Antrag und Entscheidungsfindung der Ethikkommission Lübeck. Rechtsmedizin, 9 (3), 107-111.

Office of Science and Technology (OST), 1997. Memorandum submitted by the Office of Science and Technology (10 March 1997) (CLE 7). In STC, Fifth report of sessions 1996-1997 - the cloning of animals from adult cells - Vol. II minutes of evidence and appendices. London: The Stationery Office, 42-47.

Rein, M. and Schön, D., 1993. Reframing policy discourse. In Fischer, F. and Forester, J., eds. The argumentative turn in policy analysis and planning. Durham: Duke University Press, 145-166.

ReproKult, 2002a. Human is human. In ReproKult, eds. Reproductive medicine and genetic engineering. Women between self-determination and societal standardisation. Bonn: Bundeszentrale für gesundheitliche Aufklärung, 130-132.

ReproKult, 2002b. Position on embryo and embryonic stem cell research. In ReproKult, eds. Reproductive medicine and genetic engineering. Women between self-determination and societal standardisation. Bonn: Bundeszentrale für gesundheitliche Aufklärung, 137-138.

ReproKult, 2002c. Position on preimplantation genetic diagnosis (PGD). In ReproKult, eds. Reproductive medicine and genetic engineering. Women between self-determination and societal standardisation. Bonn: Bundeszentrale für gesundheitliche Aufklärung, 135-136.

ReproKult, 2002d. Forum 7: ethics or politics? In ReproKult, eds. Reproductive medicine and genetic engineering. Women between self-determination and societal standardisation. Bonn: Bundeszentrale für gesundheitliche Aufklärung, 110-120.

Royal Society, 2004. Science in society report. London: Royal Society.

Schmidt, U., 2001. Gesundheitspolitik des Vertrauens. Erstes Pressegespräch mit der Bundesgesundheitsministerin Ulla Schmidt. 31 January.

http://www.bmg.bund.de/deu/gra/aktuelles/reden/bmgs/index_2763.cfm [Accessed 1 February 2005].

Schröder, G., 2000. Der neue Mensch. Beitrag zur Gentechnik von Bundeskanzler Gerhard Schröder für die Wochenzeitung Die Woche. Die Woche, 20 December 2000.

Science and Technology Committee (STC), 1997a. Fifth report of sessions 1996-1997—the cloning of animals from adult cells - Vol. I, report. London: The Stationery Office.

Science and Technology Committee (STC), 1997b. Fifth report of sessions 1996-1997— the cloning of animals from adult cells - Vol. II, minutes of evidence and appendices. London: The Stationery Office.

Sexton, S., 2000. How to talk about cloning without talking about cloning. Public discourse in the UK [online]. Interdepartmental Centre for Ethics in the Sciences and Humanities, University of Tübingen. Available from: http://www.thecornerhouse.org.uk/item.shtml?x=52016 [Accessed 7 April 2010].

Spaemann, R., 2001. Gezeugt, nicht gemacht. Die verbrauchende Embryonenforschung ist ein Anschlag auf die Menschenwürde. In Geyer, C., ed. Biopolitik. Die Positionen. Frankfurt: edition suhrkamp, 41-50.

Südwest Presse Ulm, 2000. Menschen dürfen nicht zu Objekten werden. Interview with Heinz Krus, spokesman of the citizen initiative against the Bioethics Convention. Südwest Presse Ulm, 3 February 2000. Available from: http://www.fuente.de/bioethik/swp_000203.htm [Accessed 2 August 2010].

Tolmein, O., 1998. Ein Recht auf fehlerfreie Babys? Gen-ethischer Informationsdienst GID, 125/126, 57-58.

Wilkie, T., and Graham, E., 2001. Power without responsibility. Media portrayals of British science. In Klotzko, A.J., ed. The cloning sourcebook. Oxford: University Press, 135-150.

Wynne, B., 2001. Creating public alienation: expert cultures of risk and ethics on GMOs. In Science as culture, 10 (4), 445-481.

ZES, Zentrale Ethikkommission für Stammzellforschung, 2009. Siebter Tätigkeitsbericht nach Inkrafttreten des Stammzellgesetzes für den Zeitraum von 01.12.2008 bis 30.11.2009. Available from: http://www.rki.de/cln_178/nn_207098/DE/Content/Gesund/Stammzellen/ZES/Taetigkeitsberichte/7-taetigkeitsbericht,templateId=raw,propertypublicationFile.pdf/7-taetigkeitsbericht.pdf [Accessed 17 March 2010].

Post-apocalyptic discourse and the new modesty: governing preimplantation genetic diagnosis in the UK

KATHRIN BRAUN AND SUSANNE SCHULTZ

This chapter is based on research from a collaborative European research project (PaGanInI) on new forms of governing in a variety of issue areas related to nature and/or the body.[1] These issue areas are characterized by high levels of risk, uncertainty, controversy, and public concern and the project began from the hypothesis that the structure of these issues would pose considerable challenges to conventional, classical modernist forms of government. The classical or high modernist paradigm of policy making, as understood by the PaGanInI team, is predicated on the assumption that society and social action can be governed from the centre, namely from well-defined, constitutional government bodies, and that the state, clearly delimited against society, can rely on synoptic, universally valid and politically neutral expert knowledge in order to plan and control social processes (Gottweis/Braun 2007, Hajer/Wagenaar 2003, Scott 1998). High modernist statecraft, however, is confronted with a series of challenges arising from matters of risk and uncertainty, public concerns and claims to public par-

---

1 PaGanInI (Participatory Governance and Institutional Innovation), 6th EU Framework Programme, contract no. CIT2-CT-2004-505791 (http://www.paganini-project.net/).

ticipation, and a dwindling belief in the neutrality and authority of scientific expertise. Responding to these challenges, we supposed, would involve institutional modification or innovation (Gottweis/Braun 2007, Gottweis/Braun/Haila/Hajer et al 2008). The project set out to explore several connected empirical questions (The Paganini Project 2007). Have these challenges indeed prompted innovations in government? If so, which forms of government and steering have emerged? To what extent do they accommodate uncertainty, give room to the contested character of knowledge, and take public concerns seriously? Are they more fluid, open, de-centralized and participatory?

The research presented here is based on a study conducted within the framework of the PaGanInI project on the politics of genetic testing and the controversies surrounding it since the 1980s in Germany and the UK. Our findings here with respect to the central research questions were mixed. Rather than confirming whole-heartedly that high modernist statecraft has been superseded by new, innovative, more participatory, flexible and decentralized forms of government in response to the new challenges, we found two things: first, in this field, classical modernist forms of government largely endured in Germany, while new and considerably different forms have emerged in the UK. The German situation is still characterized by a focus on the law and the constitution as the main instruments of regulation, emphasizing fixed, legally binding principles such as human dignity, and confirming the decision-making authority of the Parliament and, always in the background, the Constitutional Court. In addition, conventional advisory bodies play an important role and their members are still largely constructed as experts, and not as laypeople or members of the public. The main institutional innovation within this mode of governing was the inclusion of new *types* of experts, such as philosophers or sociologists in addition to traditional types, such as scientists, lawyers and physicians. Another innovation in this field in Germany is the institutionalization of ethical deliberation.[2] Experiments with formal state-sponsored public participation, such as citizen conferences and youth conferences, however, remain rudimentary (Braun/Schultz 2009). At the same time, in Germany, the predominantly classical modern mode of government was, at least for a period,

---

2 For a more detailed account on the German bioethics debate see Braun 2005; Braun/Moore/Herrmann/Könninger 2010; and Herrmann 2009.

accompanied by a comparatively intense and polarized public debate, particularly on the issue of preimplantation genetic diagnosis (PGD).[3]

Second, and this will be the main topic of this chapter, the post-classical forms of governing that have arisen in this issue area in the UK since the 1980s have their own ambiguities that are worth scrutinizing. We found that in the UK a pragmatic, flexible, and proceduralized mode of government has developed that is based on processes of negotiation, internal deliberation and public participation. It is characterized by incremental decision-making, elastic and temporary categories rather than general, fixed rules, an orientation towards specific contexts and personal values and emotions rather than universal principles, and an emphasis on public participation as a means of mapping values, arguments and concerns outside the expert world. The type of knowledge that proves useful within this mode of governing is generated through processes of deliberation and interpretation, is context-sensitive, and refers strongly to values and emotions. Compared to classical modernist statecraft, both the forms and the sources of useful policy knowledge have expanded and a series of dualisms have become blurred or lost significance: between scientific and non-scientific experts, between experts and laypeople, rationality and subjectivity, or universal and context-specific validity. In addition to these shifts, a new modesty has emerged in science policy discourse, which emphasizes the limits and the uncertainty of technoscientific knowledge rather than its truth, reliability and therefore authority. In this chapter, we argue that while there is indeed a new institutional flexibility, this flexibility ultimately promotes a quite linear development towards the normalization and proliferation of PGD. We will show that the new institutional flexibility as well as the new modesty do not undermine, but rather support a permissive approach towards the technology. If one takes a techno-optimistic stance, with

---

3   This situation of antagonistic public controversy however, did not endure. In 2010, at the time of writing this chapter, the German Federal Court of Justice (Bundesgerichtshof) had just issued a ruling that the wording of the German Embryo Protection Act would not imply a ban on PGD and that thus a physician who had practiced it had not thereby offended the law (Bundesgerichtshof 2010). Whether due to the authority of the Court or due to a change in public attitude: the German public remained strikingly silent and apparently accepted this interpretation as a fact.

individual freedom of choice reigning supreme, this is not a problem. If one takes a more critical view towards selection practices such as PGD, and appreciates public contestation on the issue, the new flexible approach gives less cause for celebration. In the following, we will examine the new institutional flexibility from this critical perspective.

To some extent, the points presented here are consistent with the theoretical framework of reflexive modernity developed by Ulrich Beck and others (Beck/Bonss/Lau 2003). Reflexive modernity scholars hold that science has lost its monopoly on legitimate knowledge and along with it the power to close debates and inform decision-making. This monopoly, they suggest, has been replaced by a multiplicity of knowledges and rationalities. The role of science, according to this analysis, is no longer to minimize uncertainty and silence controversy but to take uncertainty into account and to offer a plurality of different viewpoints. Institutional processes of self-consciously *drawing* boundaries, so goes the argument, have replaced the taken for granted existence of boundaries such as that between scientific and other rationalities. While many of these observations do apply to the issue area under study here, we feel that we need a more detailed and specific view of reflexive modernity in this context, a picture that shows more closely *how* new boundaries are drawn and decisions are made (see also Braun/Moore/Herrmann/Könninger 2010). Also, we are more skeptical about the assumption that the blurring of boundaries, dichotomies, and monopolies as such opens up space for contestation and democracy. Before we present the case study, we will briefly describe the practice of PGD.

PGD: A TECHNOLOGY OF RISK AND UNCERTAINTY

PGD is only one area of genetic testing among many, but it is arguably still the most controversial one, both in the UK and in Germany. It combines the practice of in vitro fertilization (IVF) and the application of tests for chromosomal or genetic disorders on the embryo in vitro. As such, it is one focus for the increasing number of tests for genetic—or genetically related—disorders that have been the main outcome of the Human Genome Project. Since it was launched in 1990, the Human Genome Project and ongoing genome association studies have generated an enormous expansion of knowledge. This has not yet produced a comparable expansion of therapies, but it has generated an increasing number of genetic tests. According to the Human Genome Project's website, more than a thousand tests for genetic disorders or diseases are available (Human Genome Project Information 2010). In principle, though not in practice, due to the costly and onerous procedures involved, all these tests could be applied in combination with an in vitro fertilization procedure. The purpose of such PGD is to determine which embryo is to be transferred to the woman's womb. The first birth from an embryo selected following PGD took place in 1990 in London. In this case, PGD was used for sex determination in order to select out embryos that would carry a genetic disorder linked to the X-chromosome (Handyside/Lesko/Tarín/Winston et al 1992).

During the 1990s, the number of tests for genetic disorders increased steadily. Many of the tests are for so-called low-penetrance conditions. The penetrance indicates the chance that a person who carries a certain genetic mutation will actually be afflicted by the disease. Low penetrance thus means that although carriers are estimated to have a so-called higher risk of developing the disease, it is not certain that the disease will develop. PGD, in contrast to prenatal diagnosis, which takes place during pregnancy, is still comparatively controversial. It can be used to screen out those embryos that display certain undesired genetic features or for purposes of tissue typing, resulting in a so-called savior sibling. The latter is a method to "select embryos who can provide a matched tissue donation to an existing sibling", as the British HFEA puts it (HFEA 2009a).

Genetic testing in general has been termed a risk technology in a twofold sense (Lemke 2000). On the one hand it is meant to calculate risks, such as the risk of giving birth to a baby with a genetic or chromosomal disorder or the risk of getting ill later in life. On the other, it also implies risks to users, such as the risk of being excluded from access to life insurance or private health insurance. In addition, there is the risk of misdiagnosis or erroneous interpretation of test results.[4] It is worth noticing that the term risk here refers on the one hand to the likelihood that certain undesired events, such as breast cancer, will occur. "Risk" in this sense is a matter of calculation, requiring scientific expertise. On the other hand, the term risk is also frequently used to point out negative social implications of the tech-

---

4 For erroneous interpretations of test results in case of Huntington's disease, for instance, see Ibarreta/Elles/Cassiman/Rodriguez-Cerezo et al 2004.

nology, or the possibility thereof, implications that by nature cannot be calculated by scientists. The term "social risks" mostly refers to the possibility of new forms of discrimination against people living with disabilities or people who are genetically diagnosed as having a higher "risk" to develop a disease later in life. The probability of social discrimination, however, cannot be measured or quantified by scientists. Hence, risk discourse in this field slightly differs from risk discourses in other fields, such as nuclear energy, in that it also calls for non-scientific types of knowledge. Thus, discourses about "social risks" here rather refer to the generation of non-calculable uncertainty than to "risk" in the sense of calculable probabilities that could be brought under scientific control.[5]

More fundamentally, the term risk, when applied to the individual level, tends to obfuscate matters rather than clarify them. At the level of populations, probabilistic risk calculation of, for instance, the frequency of persons developing a specific disease later in life may provide a rational base for public health policies. From the perspective of the individual concerned, however, such calculations rather bring about fundamental uncertainty. This is especially true for current scientific knowledge on so-called "multi-factorial disorders." The vast part of genetic research today goes into multi-factorial disorders common in Western societies such as heart disease, diabetes, arthritis, Alzheimer's disease, or cancer (Hopkins/Nightingale 2004, Lock 2005). These disorders are related to different types of factors such as genetic factors, epigenetic factors, social and physical environment factors, and lifestyle. In the case of multi-factorial disorders, the uncertainty of test results is high with respect to the question of whether a person will actually develop the particular disease in the future, and thus which preventative measures could be helpful for him or her. Uncertainty, here, is not due to a lack of knowledge or a plurality of diverging scientific views but is built

---

5 Note that we do not use the terms risk and uncertainty in an essentialist sense. Neither do we think that certain practices per se bring about "increased" risk or uncertainty, nor do we think that certain technologies imply *either* risks *or* uncertainties. What interests us here is only that the *discourse* on risks in the context of genetic testing to some extent describes the problem at stake in a way that calls not only for scientific experts and their instruments of calculation and control but for other types of remedies too.

into the epistemic character of the risk knowledge on an individual level (Rose/Novas 2000, Samerski 2006, Weir 1996).

THE NEW MODESTY AND ANTI-GENETIC EXCEPTIONALISM

In the 1980s and 1990s, the idea that genetic testing creates rather than removes uncertainty was emphasized mainly by critics of the technology. In recent years, however, the uncertainty of genetic knowledge has been emphasized not only by critics but also by proponents of genetic testing. Geneticists, experts or policy-makers who argue that genetic testing is a normal medical technology, that public concerns are largely unfounded and that the technology does not require specific legislation, do so by pointing to the non-deterministic character of the information provided and by de-emphasizing the efficiency of the technology. A new modesty has emerged. By new modesty we mean an approach, particularly on the part of scientists and science advocates, that emphasizes the limits of what science and technology can do and thereby seeks to dampen both optimism and concern. In particular, the new modesty is directed against anxieties that human genetics entails a new biological determinism that would reduce the individual to his or her genes and use the individual genetic make-up as a criterion for social stratification. The new modesty seeks to calm anxieties about a dystopian future in which control, surveillance, and discrimination based on genetic information will be ubiquitous. What the new modesty narrative tells us is that these concerns are unfounded since genetic knowledge is simply too uncertain to provide the technical tools of such a dystopia. In other words, genetic testing is at best useful and at worst harmless; it just provides specific medical information, that may increase the individual's range of options—with increased options meaning increased freedom to decide on different therapies or behaviors. Thus, de-emphasizing the efficiency of the technology serves as a strategy to soothe public concerns.

According to critics of genetic exceptionalism, nothing particularly distinguishes genes or genetic diagnosis from other types of medical diagnosis (Green/Botkin 2003). Therefore, they argue, there is no legally relevant difference between genetic testing and other diagnostic methods (Rothstein 2005). In that vein, a member of the Human Genetics Commission (HGC), which is a non-departmental public body set up in 2000 that advises Government on the impact of developments in human genetics, told us that many commission members distance themselves from the concept of genetic exceptionalism, explaining:

I am questioning the extent to which ethics in genetics is so very different from ethics in health care generally, because there is a point to which having this genetic exceptionalism. If you look for example at genetic data, well, it really is just about health care data—it is part of your health record, and so separating out genetic data starts to get very difficult.

Likewise, in its response to the HGC's consultation paper on the question of a national genetic databank, the pharmaceutical company GlaxoSmithKline argued that there is no rationale for treating genetic information differently and for setting up specific regulations for such data. Research into common multi-genetic diseases, they argue, requires large-scale genetic and clinical information so researchers can study possible correlations between these data. Such genetic information, they argue, is no different from other forms of biomedical data, except maybe for the case of monogenetic disorders, since it lacks predictive potential (GlaxoSmithKline n.y.). Here, the merely probabilistic character of genetic knowledge is stressed in order to avoid regulatory restrictions that might reduce the amount of available data, data which are economically interesting in that they might lead to new tests that could be marketed. Critics of genetic exceptionalism also contest the assumption that information produced by genetic tests is more personal—and accordingly more sensitive—than other information about the individual. Critics of genetic testing practices, on the other hand, have come under pressure to respond to this discursive strategy. An interviewee from Human Genetics Alert, an NGO in the UK, warns that the possibility of genetic discrimination in the future should not be underestimated, given the possibility of risk calculations on the basis of genetic testing. Thus the uncertain status of genetic knowledge itself has become a challenge to political positions on both the affirmative and the skeptical sides.

A "new modesty" type of argument often comes into play as a strategy to debunk public concerns that the proliferation of PGD would bring about a new eugenics. In this vein, the HGC, in a report that sums up its conclusions from and response to a public consultation on PGD it had undertaken previously, states that: "For practical reasons, the number of conditions for which PGD can be offered is limited and few tests can be done on the DNA extracted from a single cell taken from an embryo. In addition, there will be few embryos available for selection" (HGC 2006: 15). The Commission interpreted public concern as being essentially about the possibility of creating so-called "designer babies," meaning the use of the technology to select for traits such as intelligence or beauty, and then declared those concerns "misplaced," since they rely on a false, deterministic understanding of genetic knowledge:

> While we are still far from a full understanding of how such characteristics are transmitted to children, it is clear that very many genes are likely to be involved and there will be complex interactions between these and other developmental factors. Even if all the genes involved were to be identified, prediction of the required characteristics would remain uncertain and the limited supply of embryos available for selection would make the finding of particular gene variant combinations very unlikely (ibid. 15).

The new modesty, here, is employed in a two-step discursive strategy, first reducing public concerns to anxieties about "designer babies," thereby ignoring concerns about indirect discrimination and devaluation of people living with disabilities, and, second, declaring these—reduced—concerns to be unfounded since they get the science wrong. In a sense, the new modesty thereby reiterates what Brian Wynne and Alan Irwin have called the "deficit model," namely the idea that public concerns about problems related to science and technology are caused by a knowledge deficit about the science and would dissolve once the deficit is rectified (Irwin/Wynne 1996).

EXTRASCIENTIFIC EXPERTISE AND GOVERNMENT BY CASES AND CONDITIONS

In what follows, we take a closer look at the debates on PGD in the UK and the way the issue has been governed. PGD is still a comparatively rarely used method of genetic testing.[6] The first fertility clinics started offering PGD in 1989 and the first baby born after PGD worldwide followed in 1990. While it is legal in the UK, at least some of its applications have given rise to public concern and debate in recent years.

PGD is regulated by the Human Fertilisation and Embryology Authority (HFEA), a statutory body which, within the general framework of the HFE Act, sets criteria and standards, licenses and monitors fertility clinics and all research involving human embryos, and also initiates and conducts public consultations. HFEA members are appointed by the UK Health Minister. Although they are all experts in their fields, at least 50 percent of the members, plus the chair, must be laypersons, defined as not being medical or scientific practitioners and not decision-makers or sponsors of research in the field of biomedicine (House of Commons Science and Technology Select Committee 2005: 87). Experts in, for instance, medical law, would still count as laypersons. Thus, the HFEA has formally and explicitly incorporated the inclusion of laypeople, in this sense that includes extrascientific expertise, into the policy-making process (Moore 2009).

The HFEA licenses clinics to perform PGD and approves the use of PGD largely on a condition-by-condition basis. Clinics need a license from the HFEA to carry out PGD for a specific condition (HFEA 2010). For a small number of conditions, the HFEA only issues case-by-case licenses, that is the clinic has to apply for approval to carry out testing for that condition for a specific couple. As a general rule, conditions have to be serious in order for the practice to be approved. The list of approved conditions is continuously widening, a process that time and again gives rise to public concerns. One of the more controversial decisions by the HFEA was to approve the use of PGD in order to screen out embryos carrying the BRCA I gene, the gene that is linked, statistically, to increased susceptibility to breast cancer. In this case, the HFEA licensed the use of PGD for selecting out a disease that is not fully penetrant and also appears later in life. The authority has also approved PGD for a type of colon cancer and a type of

---

6   The HFEA has granted licenses to eight clinics to carry out PGD. Between 2002 and 2003, 155 PGD cycles were performed in these clinics (HFEA 2005b). The largest of them, the Guy's and St. Thomas NHS Foundation Trust, conducted 330 PGD cycles from 1997 to 2005, resulting in 85 babies born (Lashwood 2006).

eye cancer which affect people in childhood or at young adult age but are also not fully penetrant. For these diseases, effective treatments are available. In fact, the BRCA1 and BRCA2 genes, commonly known as the familial breast cancer genes, may serve to illustrate the point that genetic tests generate risks and uncertainties (Parthasarathy 2005). The chance of a woman with a positive test result of developing this type of cancer in the course of her life has been calculated with an increasingly lower ratio and is currently estimated at less than 70 percent—in other words: a third of those diagnosed with "the breast cancer gene" do *not* develop breast cancer. Further, a positive result does not reveal when the disease will manifest or how it will develop. A negative test result, on the other hand, does not guarantee that the woman will not develop another type of breast cancer during her lifetime. Yet, a positive test result can lead to a range of actions, from securing preventive health care and submitting to regular physical examinations to undergoing breast amputation.

In the case of PGD for purposes of tissue typing, the HFEA decides on a case-by-case basis whether to grant a license to a specific clinic to use PGD in the case of a specific couple. However, case-by-case regulation has recently come under pressure from clinics who wish to switch to condition-by-condition regulation as the mode for regulating tissue typing (King 2010). Aside from licensing and monitoring, the HFEA also plays an important role in initiating, structuring, and organizing public debates through conducting public consultations.

Thus, the government of PGD is de-centralized, incremental and involves extrascientific experts (the 50 percent laymember rule) and public participation. What is the role of knowledge within this mode of governing, and which type of knowledge is considered useful for policy- and decision-making?

BEYOND SCIENTIFIC EXPERTISE:
INTERPRETATION, EMOTIONS AND STORY TELLING

In the following section we will look at the status and the understanding of knowledge that informs the mode of governing PGD in the UK. The approach to "serious diseases" gives a good illustration of the idea of relevant knowledge in this context. As a general policy, the HFEA decided to license PGD only in cases of "serious diseases." It stipulates that "a particular genetic condition is sufficiently serious before clinics are permitted to test for that condition using preimplantation genetic diagnosis ..." (HFEA 2009b, see also Ziegler 2004). "Seriousness," thus, is the relevant concept that guides and informs policy and decision-making. Significantly, it is not a scientific concept; it does not provide a universal, science-based criterion but, on the contrary, is both derived from, and applied through, context-specific interpretations and negotiations that systematically take subjective values and emotions into account. Basing decision-making on this type of context-specific interpretation allows for an incremental expansion of applications rather than political contestation of the practice as such.

Extrascientific knowledge, here, is considered not only legitimate, but indispensable for decision-making. The concept of serious genetic disorders refers back to the 1967 Abortion Act and its amendment in 1990, which allows a woman to have an abortion at any state of the pregnancy when the fetus is affected by a "serious medical handicap," with the concept of "serious" not being defined within the Act (HGC 2004: 21). As regards the application of PGD, the concept of serious remained contentious. The policy of the HFEA was deliberately not to define or scientifically clarify it but instead to interpret it on a context-specific basis: "The seriousness of a condition," the HFEA argued, "should be a matter for discussion between the people seeking treatment and the clinical team" (HFEA & HGC 2001). This policy is analogous to that adopted by the UK Royal College of Obstetricians and Gynaecologists toward abortion on the grounds of "fetal abnormality." The Royal College suggests that "the interpretation of 'serious abnormality' should be based upon individual discussion agreed between the parents and the mother's doctor" (Royal College of Obstetricians and Gynaecologists 2008, Wahlberg 2009). At the clinical level, the decision whether or not to carry out PGD is also a matter of discussion and discretion, rather than the application of fixed principles or rules; counseling is the form that binds together discretion, discussion, and decision-making. Alison Lashwood, a consultant nurse at the largest PGD clinic in the UK, explains:

The severity of a condition—the conception of this—may vary tremendously from family to family. It is not enough just looking at a situation of a child with a genetic disorder without looking at that within the context of the family, the family experience, what has happened before, how many children this couple have (Lashwood 2006).

While the concept of serious diseases was never really defined, it was nevertheless meant to draw a line between morally acceptable and unacceptable practices, forming a barrier to "prevent it being used for frivolous or 'social' reasons, or for eugenic purposes" (HFEA & ACGT 1999: 12). Yet, the concept of serious diseases has turned out to be elastic. The HFEA has not provided a conclusive definition of the concept. Nor has it set up a conclusive list of serious diseases. Rather, the list of conditions licensed for PGD has grown continuously with the availability of new genetic tests (HFEA 2010).

This dynamic of expansion was driven by a series of highly personalized stories that circulated in the media, stories about personal suffering, hope and expectations. Such stories were particularly influential in the public controversies on the creation of so-called savior siblings and on the issue of PGD for detecting late-onset diseases. One of the stories was that of Zain Hashmi. Zain suffered from thalassemia, a genetic disorder listed by the HFEA as a "serious disease," which would justify the use of PGD in order to prevent the birth of an affected child. The HFEA approved the creation of a "savior sibling" who would serve as a tissue donor for Zain. It argued that the prospective sibling was also at risk of being affected by thalassemia and that PGD therefore served not only to select a tissue donor but also to select out affected embryos. In the later case of Charlie Whitaker, who suffered from a non-genetic disease, Diamond-Blackfan disease, future siblings were not at risk of developing the disease. The identification of a savior sibling was therefore the sole ground for using PGD, so the HFEA denied a license to the family at the time (Wasserman 2003). Later, however, the HFEA also allowed cases similar to the Whitaker case on the grounds of a priority shift: While in the beginning the (small) risk of the prospective savior sibling being born with a genetic disorder was considered more important, later the HFEA in a more contextual way ascribed a higher priority to the "welfare of the family" and their right to "reproductive choice" (Mills 2006).

The stories of "the Hashmis" or "the Whitakers" stirred enormous public attention and were widely covered by the British media. These stories were about suffering and the need for making hard choices, giving rise to countless discussions of pros and cons. They were also about the need for the expert community to show empathy toward the individuals involved in such cases. They illustrate the prominent role of ethics, emotions, stories, and personal accounts in this issue area. Stories proved to be quite powerful in the issue area of PGD in general, even when they referred not to concrete persons but to hypothetical examples. This was the case with a story about a deaf couple demanding PGD in order to select an embryo with a specific form of inherited deafness (Brecher 2006, Mills 2006)—a story evoked by nearly all our interviewees in the UK. It was widely debated in British consultation processes, signaling the potentially troubling consequences of genetic technology and the need to draw a clear line between morally acceptable and unacceptable ways of employing it. The story called for reflection and empathy and was presented as a complicated but fascinating moral dilemma, framed in terms of a conflict between reproductive autonomy on the one hand and the welfare of the child on the other. Yet there was no such case in the UK at the time. In fact, the story referred to a merely hypothetical setting originating from an article about a deaf lesbian couple in the US who planned to use artificial insemination—*not* PGD—to select a sperm donor with a genetic condition linked to deafness (Spriggs 2002). It was not until 2008 that a couple did apply for PGD in the UK for the purpose of having a deaf baby (Gray 2008). Eventually, the story was incorporated into clause 14(9) of the revised Human Fertilisation and Embryology Bill in 2008, stipulating that embryos known to have a genetic abnormality "must not be preferred to those that are not known to have such an abnormality," a provision designed to rule out the selection through PGD of, for instance, a deaf child.

PUBLIC PARTICIPATION, EDUCATION AND KNOWLEDGE PRODUCTION

Extrascientific truths—such as the family situation, the welfare of the future child, the fears and hopes of family members, the couple's assessment of how "serious" the disease is *to them*—play an integral part in the decision-making process. In order to establish these extrascientific, social, and personal truths, the discussion within the triangle of applicant, doctor, and the authority forms a crucial site of the governing process. Governing this issue is thus highly proceduralized: on the one hand, governing devices (the list of "serious conditions") continuously incorporate the process of technoscientific development; on the other hand, key criteria (seriousness) are being proceduralized by being submitted to interpretation and discussion. Within this flexible and pragmatic style of government, a permissive stance towards technoscientific development and a rather extrascientific approach of referring to context, meaning, and interpretation as mechanisms of government are not mutually exclusive or even opposed to one another. One could understand institutionalized public participation procedures as another device for procedural government, in that they also serve to discuss the meaning of a certain practice and to establish the range of adequate feelings, attitudes, and values at stake, only on a larger scale. Javier Lezaun and Linda Soneryd (2007) regard formal participation exercises as "technologies of elicitation," which seems particularly appropriate in the issue area of genetic testing since public consultations serve not least to establish which feelings, attitudes, and values people—who are also potential users—hold towards this practice (Braun/Schultz 2009).

Formal public participation arrangements are well established in UK policy making, specifically in the field of biomedicine and biotechnology. Genetic testing in general as well as PGD in particular has been subject to a series of public consultations since the late 1990s. Even though PGD is generally accepted by the British public, it still "pushes some very sensitive buttons of some individuals, on both sides," as one of our interviewees put it. It has given rise to various debates within expert communities, government institutions, the media, and civil society, evoking concerns about the creation of "designer babies," sex selection, a "slippery slope" towards eugenics, and the moral status of the embryo. It is part of the remit of government advisory bodies or authorities such as the HFEA, the Advisory Committee on Genetic Testing (ACGT, 1996-1999) or the HGC to take up, respond to, structure and organize such debates through formal participatory arrangements. The main instrument of such participation in the UK is a public consultation. A public consultation in the UK is a means of policy-making in which typically a government department or a regulatory body such as the HFEA writes a consultation paper, which includes information about the issue at stake as well as a set of questions or points to discuss. This document is published and circulated among different addressees with the request to provide comments or opinions, and a report is then usually drawn up incorporating these comments. The authority is free to decide *which* conclusions to draw from these consultations.

From 1999 to 2001, the HFEA, together with the Advisory Committee on Genetic Testing, conducted a public consultation on PGD (HFEA & ACGT 1999), which was later concluded by the HFEA and the HGC. In 2002–03, the HFEA conducted a public consultation on the issue of sex selection (HFEA 2003) and in 2005–06 did one on PGD for late-onset genetic conditions (HFEA 2005a). The HGC also performed a public consultation relating to PGD, on genetics and reproductive decision-making, in 2004–06 (HGC 2004, 2006). The consultation on PGD mainly focused on the question of which rules and criteria should govern the HFEA's licensing policy regarding the technology. The consultation paper suggested putting in place provisions to rule out frivolous or eugenic applications (HFEA & ACGT 1999: 12). The majority of respondents agreed, preferring that PGD should be used only for highly predictive serious disorders, not complex multifactorial disorders (HFEA & HGC 2001: 20). Two more controversial issues included licensing PGD for the creation of so-called savior siblings and for detecting late-onset diseases such as Huntington disease. After its public consultations on the issue of sex selection (HFEA 2003) and on PGD for late-onset genetic conditions (HFEA 2005a), the HFEA announced it would conduct another consultation on the issue of savior siblings. This consultation, however, never happened. Nevertheless, in the following years the HFEA did license uses of PGD that would not fall into the category of preventing "highly predictive serious disorders" and that the majority of respondents to former consultations had not approved, such as tissue typing in the case of the Hashmi family and PGD for detecting disorders that are not fully penetrant. In the case of low-penetrance conditions, the HFEA did start a consultation process on this specific issue—yet only after having already issued the license to use PGD for a type of inherited eye cancer that is not fully penetrant (ibid.). Hence, public consultations may generate knowledge about prevailing views and value judgments in the public, but the authority is by no means bound by the results of a consultation.

Overall, formal public participation arrangements in the field of genetic testing take place within a fragmented, sophisticated, non-antagonistic constellation in which techno-skeptical concerns are not dominant but are still subliminally present. By non-antagonistic constellation we mean a situation that is not characterized by an adversarial confrontation between two opposing camps that take diametrically opposed views on the issue and strive to defeat the other. Rather, techno-skeptical arguments, in this constellation, have been disconnected from an antagonistic pro-and-con constellation. The focus of such debates has shifted toward the different pros and cons and the specific conditions of acceptability of certain applications of genetic testing and away from the big visions, whether splendid or scary, of a geneticized future society. This has not always been the case. In the 1980s, feminist and disability rights groups developed a techno-skeptical discourse toward genetic testing and genetic engineering in general (Schultz/Braun/Griessler 2007). Over the past two to three decades, the dominant discursive frames have shifted from comprehensive, long-term euphoric or apocalyptical visions to dispersed, pragmatic, post-euphoric, and post-apocalyptic forms of discourse (ibid.). Nevertheless, although the debate has been redirected toward a more post-apocalyptic and post-euphoric framing, there are still moments of controversy, unease, and concern. This is especially the case with PGD. However, concerns are fragmented, referring to certain applications such as the creation of savior siblings, sex selection, and to some extent the use of PGD in cases of late-onset and/or lower penetrance genetic disorders. Furthermore, when more fundamental oppositional arguments come up, they tend to be discredited as being uninformed and irrational and excluded from the range of acceptable and important feelings.

The main purposes of such participatory arrangements, we would argue, are knowledge production and education, rather than political deliberation and decision-making. Public consultations should not be mistaken for referenda, as the former chair of the HFEA, Dame Suzi Leather, made perfectly clear. "Instead", she said, "we want to understand why people feel worried or enthusiastic about this research in order to help us make a judgment about the best way to proceed" (HFEA 2007). Thus, these arrangements may provide the authority or the government with information about people's attitudes about human genetics and the prevailing views and value judgments among the public, but the authority is by no means bound by these consultations. It can draw conclusions from them but it is free to decide *which* conclusions.

EXCURSUS: EXPORTING THE MODEL TO EUROPE?

In 2004, the European Commission published a report on "25 recommendations on the ethical, legal and social implications of genetic testing" (European Commission 2004), presenting the results of a multidisciplinary Expert Group that had been invited by the EU Commission to discuss the topic of genetic testing over a period of one year.[7] Among the expert members was Alastair Kent, member of the HGC and the director of the Genetic Interest Group in the UK. The latter is an interest group that represents a number of patient organizations, which in turn represent people affected by genetic disorders. The report exemplifies quite neatly the nexus between genetic testing as technology of risk and uncertainty, the new modesty, the need for public participation as a means of knowledge production, and an overall non-antagonistic setting, which is why we will briefly discuss it here.

The report assumes that public concern is motivated by the perception that genetic testing is somehow related to the history of eugenics. This concern, they say, is "understandable" but "inappropriate" (ibid. 11). From this, the report derives the recommendation that

> ... in order to track the evolution of public perception of genetic testing and to identify issues of future debate: further research on ethical and social perceptions of genetic testing is necessary and should be promoted by the European Commission and national bodies (ibid. 11f.).

It starts from the premise that there is a lack of knowledge about genetic testing among the public and that awareness and understanding of genetic concepts has to be increased. In order to do so, they recommend that "concerted efforts to promote dialogue, education, information and debate be encouraged" (ibid. 12). Crucially, public dialogue is recommended as a proper means to achieve a twofold aim: education and knowledge production. Quite in the spirit of the "deficit model" it is assumed that the public

---

[7] The process focussed on the work of this expert group. It also included a "European Stakeholders and Citizens' Conference." However, deliberation here was limited to the debate of the ready-made 25 expert recommendations, as one of our interviewees, a member of the European Parliament, told us.

has a knowledge deficit about genetic research. This causes unfounded concerns and fears, which can be allayed by better education about the benefits of research. At the same time, dialogue will serve as a "technology of elicitation" (Lezaun/Soneryd 2007) that will generate data about the views and attitudes held by the public. That knowledge, in turn, may help science and the government to take a more proactive approach towards public concern or public unease.

However, public dialogue, as is clearly stated, has to take a non-antagonistic form, providing no room for polarized constellations:

> Participants in the dialogue should be encouraged to be open-minded, willing to listen, respectful of local cultural values, and should treat this dialogue as an exchange of opinions rather than as an opportunity for proselytising (European Commission 2004: 12).

In order to increase public awareness of the benefits arising from genetic research and genetic testing, it is imperative, they argue in the spirit of the new modesty, to set "realistic expectations as to what they can achieve" (ibid. 11f.).

Thus, the expert group is suggesting a mode of governing contested technoscientific practices that assembles some key features of the post-classical modernist approach we saw in our case study. They promote further technoscientific development and its expanded application by employing a strategy that combines the acknowledgement of scientific uncertainty with exercises of public participation as a means of elicitation and education within the confinement of a modified deficit model and a general non-antagonistic constellation.

Conclusions

Did new, post-classical modernist forms of government emerge in response to issues of risk and uncertainty? Our overall conclusion would be that, yes, we do see a pattern of governing in the issue area under study here that considerably differs from the classical modernist pattern. It is characterized by a nexus between a new scientific modesty that deliberately accounts for the uncertainty of scientific knowledge, the incorporation of extrascientific knowledge, and formal public participation exercises within an overall non-antagonistic constellation. It has evolved within a post-euphoric and post-apocalyptic framework within which we see a new modesty among geneticists and proponents of genetic research, who tend to de-emphasize the distinctiveness of genetic knowledge and its potential implications. Within this framework, debate on PGD in the UK has focused on the acceptability of different applications rather than on the technology in general. There is clearly a new emphasis on public participation and a proliferation of formal state-sponsored public participation exercises. These formal public participation arrangements, we have argued, can be understood as means of education and knowledge production. They form devices of procedural government, serving to discuss the meaning of a certain practice and to establish the feelings and attitudes toward it and the values at stake. As such, they form part of an overarching pragmatic, flexible, and procedural mode of governing, ranging from counseling processes among patients, clinics and the authority, via the HFEA's internal deliberation processes, to processes of debate organized through public consultations. This mode of governing is characterized by incremental decisions rather than by general rules, elastic and temporary categories rather than fixed ones, regulatory bodies rather than parliament, and an emphasis on personal experiences, values, and emotions rather than universal principles. Criteria for decision-making are context-specific and based on personal meaning ("What does it mean for this family to have a child with a disposition for this disease?") rather than scientific truth ("Is this a serious disease?"). Policy-making and decision-making, here, draw strongly on extrascientific resources such as emotions, context-specific deliberations and interpretations.

In effect, this flexible, procedural mode of government is permissive and open to a gradual expansion of approved technoscientific practices. Hence, even if we see a new post-classical modernist paradigm emerging, it does not per se allow more space for political contestations, since these features are firmly entrenched in maintaining an overall non-antagonistic constellation. Within this pragmatic and proceduralized mode of government, a permissive, pro-technoscience stance is compatible with the acknowledgement of uncertainty and the incorporation of extrascientific actors and forms of knowledge.

References

Beck, Ulrich/Bonss, Wolfgang/Lau, Christoph (2003): "The theory of reflexive modernization", in: Theory, Culture and Society 20(1), pp. 1-33.
Braun, Kathrin (2005): "Not just for experts. The public debate on reprogenetics in Germany", in: Hastings Center Report 35(3), pp. 42-49.
Braun, Kathrin/Moore, Alfred/Herrmann, Svea L./Könninger, Sabine (2010): "Ethical reflection must always be measured", in: Science, Technology & Human Values 35(6), pp. 839-864.
Braun, Kathrin/Schultz, Susanne (2009): "'...a certain amount of engineering involved': constructing the public in participatory governance arrangements", in: Public Understanding of Science 19(4), pp. 403-419.
Brecher, Bob (2006): "What's wrong in eliminating handicap?", paper presented at the symposium Ethical and legal issues at the beginning of life: debating 'designer babies', Middlesex University London, 2 February 2006.
Bundesgerichtshof (2010): "Die Präimplantationsdiagnostik zur Entdeckung schwerer genetischer Schäden des extrakorporal erzeugten Embryos ist nicht strafbar", Mitteilung der Pressestelle Nr. 137/2010; available at http://juris.bundesgerichtshof.de/cgi-bin/rechtsprechung/document.py?Gericht=bgh&Art=pm&pm_nummer=0137/10 (last accessed 11/30/2010).
European Commission (2004): "25 recommendations on the ethical, legal and social implications of genetic testing", Brussels: European Commission; avaliable at http://europa.eu/comm/research/conferences/2004/genetic/pdf/recommendations_en.pdf (last accessed 12/17/2009).
GlaxoSmithKline (n.y.): "Responses to the 'Whose hands on your genes?' consultation"; available at http://www.hgc.gov.uk/Client/Content_wide.asp?ContentId=425 (last accessed 2/9/2009).
Gottweis, Herbert/Braun, Kathrin (2007): Participatory governance and institutional innovation [PAGANINI], contract no. CIT2-CT-2004-505791, deliverable no. 18, final report, June 2007; available at http://www.univie.ac.at/LSG/paganini/finals_pdf/WP8_FinalReport.pdf (last accessed 11/30/2010).
Gottweis, Herbert/Braun, Kathrin/Haila, Yrjo/Hajer, Maarten et al (2008): "Participation and the new governance of life", in: BioSocieties 3(3), pp. 265-286.

Gray, Richard (2008): "Couples could win right to select deaf baby", in: The Telegraph, 4/14/2008; available at www.telegraph.co.uk/news/uknews/1584948/Couples-could-win-right-to-select-deaf-baby.html (last accessed 12/10/2010).

Green, Michael/Botkin, Jeffrey R. (2003): "Genetic exceptionalism in medicine: clarifying the differences between genetic and nongenetic tests", in: Annals of Internal Medicine 138, pp. 571-575.

Hajer, Maarten/Wagenaar, Hendrik (2003): "Introduction", in: Maarten Hajer/Henk Wagenaar (eds), Deliberative policy analysis. Understanding governance in the network society, Cambridge, UK: Cambridge University Press, pp. 1- 30.

Handyside, Alan H./Lesko, John G./Tarín, Juan J./Winston, Robert M.L. et al (1992): "Birth of a normal girl after in vitro fertilization and preimplantation diagnostic testing for cystic fibrosis", in: New England Journal of Medicine 327(13), pp. 905-909.

Herrmann, Svea Luise (2009): Policy debates on reprogenetics. The problematization of new research in Great Britain and Germany, Frankfurt a.M.: Campus.

HFEA (2003): Sex selection: choice and responsibility in human reproduction consultation document; available at http://www.hfea.gov.uk/en/1511.html#sex_selection (last accessed 4/8/2009).

— (2005a): Choices and boundaries. Should people be able to select embryos free from an inherited susceptibility to cancer? Consultation paper, November 2005; available at http://www.hfea.gov.uk/cps/rde/xbcr/hfea/Choices_Boundaries.pdf (last accessed 11/30/2010).

— (2005b): Press release: "HFEA announce new process to speed up applications for embryo screening. 19 January 2005"; available at http://www.hfea.gov.uk/697.html (last accessed 11/30/2010).

— (2007): Press release: "Should we allow the creation of human/animal embryos? 26 April 2007"; available at http://www.hfea.gov.uk/467.html (last accessed 11/30/2010).

— (2009a): Review of preimplantation tissue typing; available at http://www.hfea.gov.uk/515.html (last accessed 12/3/2010).

— (2009b): Pre-implantation genetic diagnosis; available at http://www.hfea.gov.uk/preimplantation-genetic-diagnosis.html#3 (last accessed 12/10/2010).

— (2010): PGD conditions licensed by the HFEA; available at http://www.hfea.gov.uk/cps/hfea/gen/pgd-screening.htm (last accessed 11/30/2010).

HFEA & ACGT (1999): Consultation document on preimplantation genetic diagnosis; available at http://www.hfea.gov.uk/cps/rde/xbcr/hfea/PGD_document.pdf (last accessed 11/30/2010).

HFEA & HGC (2001): Outcome of the public consultation on preimplantation genetic diagnosis; available at http://www.hfea.gov.uk/cps/rde/xbcr/SID-3F57D79B-FEB79DDD/hfea/PGD_outcome.pdf (last accessed 11/30/2010).

HGC (2004): Human Genetics Commission: choosing the future: genetics and reproductive decision making; available at http://www.hgc.gov.uk/UploadDocs/DocPub/Document/ChooseFuturefull.pdf (last accessed 11/30/2010).

— (2006): Making babies: reproductive decisions and genetic technologies; available at http://www.hgc.gov.uk/UploadDocs/DocPub/Document/Making%20Babies%20Report%20-%20final%20pdf.pdf (last accessed 11/30/2010).

Hopkins, Paul/Nightingale, Michael M. (2004): "Risk management and the commercialization of human genetic testing in the UK", in: Maureen McKelvey/Annika Rickne/Jens Laage-Hellman (eds), The economic dynamics of biotechnologies, Cheltenham: Edwards Elgar, pp. 135-166.

House of Commons Science and Technology Select Committee (2005): Human reproductive technologies and the law, London: The Stationery Office.

Human Genome Project Information (2010): Gene testing; available at http://www.ornl.gov/sci/techresources/Human_Genome/medicine/genetest.shtml (last accessed 12/17/2009).

Ibarreta, Dolores/Elles, Robert/Cassiman Jean-Jacques/Rodriguez-Cerezo et al (2004): "Towards quality assurance and harmonization of genetic testing services in the European Union", in: Nature Biotechnology 22, pp. 1230-1235.

Irwin, Alan/Wynne, Brian (1996): Misunderstanding science? Cambridge: Cambridge University Press.

King, David (2010): "The case-by-case regulation", in: BioNews 451, pp.?

Lashwood, Allison (2006): "Preimplantation genetic diagnosis: designing babies or a useful clinical service?", speech at the symposium Ethical and legal issues at the beginning of life: debating 'designer babies', Middlesex University London, 2 February 2006.

Lemke, Thomas (2000): "Die Regierung der Risiken. Von der Eugenik zur genetischen Gouvernementalität", in: Ulrich Bröckling/Susanne Krasmann/Thomas Lemke (eds), Gouvernementalität der Gegenwart. Studien zur Ökonomisierung des Sozialen, Frankfurt a.M.: Suhrkamp, pp. 227-264.

Lezaun, Javier/Soneryd, Linda (2007): "Consulting citizens: technologies of elicitation and the mobility of publics", in: Public Understanding of Science 16(3), pp. 279-297.

Lock, Margaret (2005): "Eclipse of the gene and the return of divination", in: Current Anthropology 46(Supplement, December), pp. 47-60.

Mills, Peter (2006): "Regulating preimplantation diagnosis: a case study in moral and legal orienteering", paper presented at the symposium Ethical and legal issues at the beginning of life: debating 'designer babies', Middlesex University London, 2 February 2006.

Moore, Alfred (2009): "Public bioethics and public engagement: the politics of 'proper talk'", in: Public Understanding of Science 19(2), pp. 197-211.

The Paganini Project (2007): The PaGanInI booklet: participatory governance and institutional innovation. The new politics of life. A summary of the PaGanInI project: Department of Political Science, University of Vienna; available at http://www.univie.ac.at/LSG/paganini/output.htm (last accessed 11/30/2010).

Parthasarathy, Shobita (2005): "Architectures of genetic medicine: comparing genetic testing for breast cancer in the USA and UK", in: Social Studies of Science 35(1), pp. 5-40.

Rose, Nikolas/Novas, Carlos (2000): "Genetic risk and the birth of the somatic individual", in: Economy and Society 29(4), pp. 485-513.

Rothstein, Markus A. (2005): "Genetic exceptionalism & legislative pragmatism", in: The Hastings Center Report 35(4), pp. 27-33.Royal College of Obstetricians and Gynaecologists (2008): Q&A: Abortion for fetal abnormality and sydromatic conditions indicated by cleft lip and/or palate—the O&Q perspective; available at http://www.rcog.org.uk/what-we-do/campaigning-and-opinions/briefings-and-qas-/human-fertilisation-and-embryology-bill/abort (last accessed 11/30/2010).

Samerski, Silja (2006): "The unleashing of genetic terminology: how genetic counselling mobilizes for risk management", in: New Genetics and Society 25(2), pp. 197-208.
Schultz, Susanne/Braun, Kathrin/Griessler, Erich (2007): Work package 3_ The governance of genetic testing. A non-antagonistic setting, "authentic publics" and moments of unease; available at http://www.univie.ac.at/LSG/paganini/finals_pdf/WP3_FinalReport.pdf (last accessed 11/30/2010).
Scott, James C. (1998): Seeing like a state: how certain schemes to improve the human condition have failed, New Haven: Yale University Press.
Spriggs, M. (2002): "Lesbian couple create a child who is deaf like them", in: Journal for Medical Ethics 28, p. 283.
Wahlberg, Ayö (2009): "Serious disease as kinds of living", in Ayö Wahlberg/Susanne Bauer (eds), Contested categories: life sciences in society, Aldershot: Ashgate, pp. 89-112.
Wasserman, David (2003): "Having one child to save another. A tale of two families", in: Philosophy and Public Policy Quarterly 23(1), pp. 21-27.
Weir, Lorna (1996): "Recent developments in the government of pregnancy", in: Economy and Society 25(3), pp. 373-392.
Ziegler, Uta (2004): Präimplantationsdiagnostik in England und Deutschland. Ethische, rechtliche und praktische Probleme, Frankfurt a.M.: Campus.

Is everything in good health?
From bio to nano—the proliferation of governmental ethics in France

SABINE KÖNNINGER

"Ethics" is booming. Today issues such as abortion, preimplantation genetic diagnosis, organ donation, or in vitro fertilization are debated primarily in terms of ethics. It seems self-evident that issues in the so-called life sciences are inevitably "ethical." "Ethics" seems to be inherent in biotechnology and biomedicine. The more the developments in the life sciences advance, the more ethical problems and questions there seem to be. The language of ethics has become an important medium for discussions about such issues. Conflicts appear in terms of ethics, and governmental decisions make reference to "ethics." This development is accompanied by an increasing expertise concerning ethics and a wave of institutionalization. Since the beginning of the 1980s, the emergence of a multitude of government-sponsored or -initiated ethical institutions and procedures in the policy fields of biotechnology and biomedicine have become observable, mainly in Western societies. As in France, theses institutions usually do not have the task of providing a system for social/political limitations or regulating technoscientific development. Through recommendations and opinions as well as the inclusion of the public, they have the task of debating "ethical aspects" of research and practices in the life sciences and to inform politics as well as the public about how to deal with biomedicine and biotechnology in "ethically" justified ways (Herrmann/Könninger 2008: 205).

Not only have national ethics committees or ethics councils emerged at the interface of politics, sciences, and the public, but hearings or public opinion polls on "ethical questions" as well as citizen conferences or public debates have been carried out.

However, there is a process that goes beyond linking "ethics" with biotechnology and biomedicine. As discourses on nanotechnology[1] in France show, not only have the number of publicly sponsored procedures and bodies increased, but so have the issues they handle. The French national ethics committee discussed nanotechnology in 2007, and in 2009–10, the French government organized public debates on "ethical questions" of nanotechnologies across the country (CCNE 2007; Commission nationale du débat public 2009: 5). Concerning France, one can speak of a proliferation of "ethics" in other policy fields, often through the same governmental institutions, as the example of the French national ethics committee, *Comité consultatif national d'éthique pour les sciences de la vie et de la santé* (National Consultative Ethics Committee on Health and Life Sciences, CCNE) shows. If a committee on "health" and "the life sciences" examines nanotechnologies, it implies that more and more issues are framed in terms of ethics and therefore are subsumed under life science and health discourses. In a nutshell, it means that nanotechnologically treated car paint or self-cleaning windows are debated within the same framework as preimplantation genetic diagnosis or organ donation. It seems that "ethics" is not a question of which technological issues are discussed, but a question of *how* to discuss them. But how does an issue become an "ethical" one? And with respect to scientific governance,[2] what are the implications of utilizing the same discursive framework?

---

1   The term nanotechnology includes the biomedical and biotechnological sectors, but also energy technology, environmental technology, information technology, the food, cosmetics and textile sectors, as well as the military. For an overview of fields in which nanotechnology is applied, see Jömann/Ach 2006.
2   Following Alan Irwin, the concept of scientific governance used here refers to the government of technoscientific development on the one hand, and to governing science-society relations on the other (Irwin 2006).

From the "Magistère Bioéthique" to the "Magistère Nanoéthique"?

Making reference to Michel Foucault, the French sociologist and political scientist Dominique Memmi calls the French CCNE's way of governing "magistère bioéthique." According to her, it is a kind of government that focuses on self-control accompanied by expertise (Memmi 2005). Memmi situates the "magistère bioéthique" in a broader context of what she calls delegated biopolitics (Memmi 2003a: 289): a biopolitical mechanism that is characterized by a transformation from disciplining the population to an accompanying self-government of the individual. Governmental spheres of action are increasingly shifted or "delegated" to the responsibility of the individual without the state backing out entirely. This new government is concentrated especially on the government of bodily conduct, of the "bio" or "soma." This "bioindividuation" means balancing bodily conditions, calculating risks, and evaluating the costs of one's own health and its improvement (Memmi 2005). The conduct of this kind of self-government does not take place via bans or punishment but through a certain kind of expert-led type of speech, such as the ethical speech of the CCNE that stimulate individual and "rational" self-control (Memmi 2003b).

In addition to Memmi's work on the CCNE's type of government, recent research by Braun et al on "governmental ethics regimes"[3] in the context of scientific governance in Germany, France, and Great Britain focuses on the frame of "proper ethics talk" (Braun/Herrmann/Moore/Könninger 2010a; 2010b; Herrmann/Könninger 2008). From the perspective of Braun et al, "ethics" provides the frame for an individual, self-reflecting, and measured way of speaking and thinking concerning one's own bodily existence and scientific development. This kind of thinking and speaking takes place via the nature of the conduct of participants in "ethical" deliberations and through the formation of a certain speaker position. A "no go" within the ethics frame is the questioning of scientific development or arguing in an antagonistic way. In this sense, "ethics" shapes the frame for the production of discourse rather than providing a substantial normative course of

---

3 Governmental ethics is a modification of Susan Kelly's term "public bioethics" that stands in contrast to academic, clinical, or corporate bioethics (Kelly 2003).

action (Braun/Herrmann/Moore/Könninger 2010a; 2010b: 515; Herrmann/ Könninger 2008).

The study of governmental ethics regimes as well as Dominique Memmi's analysis took place against the background of the fact that ethical institutions and procedures deal with matters of biomedicine and biotechnology. As the CCNE worked on issues that focus on human "bodies," such as organ donation, preimplantation genetic diagnostics, or stem cell research, one can say that up to that point these issues were explicitly framed as "ethical." The newest developments in France, that is the proliferation of "ethics" in the field of nanotechnology mostly by governmental bodies and procedures that once were limited to biomedical and biotechnological issues, allow me to examine the extent to which the "governmental ethics regime" and the "magistère bioéthique" expand to new fields with great flexibility, or whether one even has to think of an evolving "magistère nanoéthique" or not. Based on the results of Memmi and Braun et al and on the observation of the proliferation of "ethics" in France, I will discuss the thesis that "ethics" can be easily extended to nanotechnological issues because it does not provide a substantial normative framework but a frame for "flexible" discourse organization. In the following, I will first concentrate on the question of how biotechnological and nanotechnological issues arc framed as ethical issues. When did the language of ethics in bio- and nanotechnological discourses emerge and what has been problematized? And second, what does "ethics" mean in these contexts? Do the characteristics of the "magistère bioéthique" and the "governmental ethics regime"—the concentration on the management of one's own health through ethical speech, the formation of a certain speaker position, and, along with it, the indisputability of ongoing research—apply just for the ethical framing of biotechnological and biomedical issues or for nanotechnological issues as well? These questions will be pursued with regard to one ethics institution in France: the CCNE. The study[4] is based on an analysis of key documents, such as constituting documents, institutional reports, or position papers; participant observations of public meetings; and expert interviews with

---

4   The study is part of the research project Converging Institutions funded by the Volkswagen Foundation and held at the Karlsruhe Institute of Technology, Germany (funding initiative Innovation processes in economy and society, Grant no II/83 568).

(former) members of the national ethics committee held in the period between 2005 and 2010.5 6

"ETHICS" AS A FRAME FOR INTERPRETATION

Analyses in the social or political sciences about the way science policy deals with "ethical" issues are to be found mainly in discourses in the fields of biomedicine or agricultural biotechnology. Susan Kelly thinks that conflicts in science and technology in the US occur within a framework of increasingly moralized politics. She shows how public bioethics bodies work as "border guards" in the relationship between politics, science, and ethics (Kelly 2003). However, when and why were these public bodies set up and what do the various actors consider to be ethical issues in "moralized politics"? Here, an example is given by Les Levidow and Susan Carr, who examine ethical issues in the policy field of agricultural biotechnology (Levidow/Carr 1997). The two authors elaborate on which ethical issues are marginalized by which players or downplayed in the policy process in the UK and at the European level.

With regard to my study, assuming that there are "ethical issues" or "moralized politics" does not explain the increasing prominence and meaning of *explicit* "ethics" in politics and the shift from bio- to nanotechnological issues often practiced by the same institutions. Sociopolitical issues imply normative questions without explicitly referring to ethics: the nuclear power conflicts of the 1970s and 1980s in Europe, for example, were also marked by conflicts of values such as responsibility towards fu-

---

5   The statements gained by the interviews and participant observations and cited in this article are translated by the author (SK).
6   Partly, documents on "bioethics" in France could be obtained by the research project titled Ethical Governance? conducted at the University of Hanover, Germany (2004-2006). The project analyzed the "governmental ethics regimes" in Germany, France and GB, referring to a range of institutions, discourses, and practices initiated or supported by governmental institutions and directed at linking ethical considerations to policy-making, especially in the field of biomedicine and biotechnology (Braun/Hermann/Könninger/Moore 2008; 2009; 2010a; 2010b; Herrmann/Könninger 2008).

ture generations. No ethics institutions were established, however, and controversies were not debated in terms of ethics but in terms of risk. In order to trace when and how nano- and biotechnological problems become framed as ethical issues, when and why the language of ethics emerges, I use the term ethics in a nominalist sense. That is, I will not define what ethics is or is not, but will try to understand what is meant by ethics in a particular context and by the actors involved (Herrmann/Könninger 2008; Könninger 2009; 2010). Instead of understanding "ethics" as inherent to biotechnological issues, methodologically I will consider ethics as a frame (Rein/Schön 1993: 153). My analysis is based on the assumption that "ethics" provides a frame for interpreting a situation or issue, determines what is problematic about it, and inherently suggests ways to deal with, think, and speak about it (speaker position). With a Foucauldian understanding of discourse, I do not take the "ethical character" of scientific issues for granted but instead consider "ethics" as a historical form of problematization[7] that has particular consequences for scientific governance (Foucault 1991: 102ff.).

THE EMERGENCE OF "ETHICS" IN BIOTECHNOLOGICAL DISCOURSES: PREVENTING CONFLICTS

In France, the language of ethics attained the level of regulatory politics within the context of debates on genetic engineering evolving within the scientific community in the 1970s.

The first ethics committees, and predecessors of the CCNE, were established as early as the mid-1970s by the *Délégation générale à la recherche scientifique*, a predecessor of the Ministry of Research (Krauss 1996), as well as by the national research institute, the *Institut national de la santé et de la recherche médicale* (Alias 1992: 129). The key events, which also apply to other countries,[8] and that were instrumental for the establishment of the CCNE, were two international conferences held in Asilomar, California, in 1973 and 1975. There, scientists discussed the risks of recombinant DNA technology (Berg/Baltimore/Boyer/Cohen et al 1974) and the

---

7   On "problematization" see Herrmann 2009.
8   Concerning the UK and Germany see Braun/Herrmann/Könninger/Moore 2008.

concept of responsibility emerged. The conferences were characterized by the awareness of the social and political responsibility of science as well as by the effort to avoid legal regulation (Krimsky 1982: 141). Although arguments around potentially undesirable or dangerous consequences of technoscientific developments were still primarily framed in terms of risks, the concept of responsibility played an important role. Furthermore, Asilomar provoked the initiation of debates in France: parallel to the Asilomar process, French scientists were organizing an international conference in Paris on "Biology and the Future Development of Humankind" (Galpérine 1976; transl. SK). One result of the conference was the founding of a scientific association, the *Mouvement de la responsabilité scientifique*, a platform for the discussion of problems with respect to scientific development and responsibility (Mouvement de la responsabilité scientifique 2005). In addition, the first ethics institutions for evaluating research projects were established. Yet, the emergence of the language of ethics—through the term responsibility—and the first French ethics committees grew out of the Asilomar process and risk discourse. Until then, the language of risks stabilized the demands of science for self-regulation and non-interference in that it framed the assessment and containment of risks as a technical matter (Evans 2002). "Risk" and "responsibility" formed a new discursive framework to reconcile the need for problematization with the effort to stabilize science's claim to self-government. This framework allowed for the coexistence of the opposing tendencies of questioning versus stabilizing scientific self-government. "Ethics" can be understood as a further framework that has its origins in the "risk and responsibility" framework, but then augmented it and to some extent eventually superseded it (Braun/Moore/Herrmann/Könninger 2010b).

A further strand where the language of ethics emerged is in the context of the anticipation of a politicized public debate about genetic technology challenging the role of science in society. Concerns about the potential of a public debate were voiced in a French report on "Life Sciences and Society" (Gros/Jacob/Royer 1979; transl. SK), which was published in the late 1970s and commissioned by Giscard d'Estaing, who was head of state at the time. The authors of the report stated that society accepted the life sciences and in particular the struggles against disease were socially accepted, in contrast to nuclear technology. They were seen as a counterbalance to the excesses of nuclear technology. But, the authors argued, conflicts did exist which could endanger the place of life sciences in society (ibid. 279ff.). On the governmental level, an analogous development to that of nuclear technology was problematized. While the conflicts on genetic technology gained attention via a debate between opponents published in the daily newspaper *Le Monde* (6/17/1975 cited by Mendel 1980: 226), and apart from that remained vital in the scientific circles of research institutes, criticism in the context of nuclear technology developed into a social movement. The latter was highlighted in the protests and demonstrations against the *Superphénix* in Malville (1976/77) (Touraine 1982). What has been thematized within the critique of nuclear technology as well as within that of genetic technology has not only been techno-skeptical elements, but also scientific decision-making, as the following example of the discourse on gene technology shows: "These manipulations concern us all. The decisions have to be taken by all" (Mendel 1980: 224; transl. SK). The report "Life Sciences and Society" illustrates that a public debate about the principles of genetic technology and above all about decision-making has been anticipated and at the same time "ethicized": "The constraints that weigh down on scientific research are increasing over time: ethical and social constraints on one side; technological and industrial obligations on the other" (Gros/Jacob/Royer 1979: 283; transl. SK). With respect to the report, the problem is framed in the language of ethics, the "ethical constraints" on the part of society. In considering these effects, the authors of the report determined that the developments and applications of the life sciences could not remain a matter for professional self-regulation in the manner of Asilomar, since the very place of the life sciences in society was being questioned. The "solution" for these "ethical constraints" and the problems for research lay in the establishment of a reflection group in dialogue: "[Dialogue] enables research to preserve a measure of freedom ... without ... losing its legitimacy and efficiency" (ibid. 282; transl. SK). In order to put this dialogue into practice, a model was proposed that for the first time resembled the later national ethics committee. It was designed to bring together scientists, politicians, and persons with various competences in a continual process of deliberation (ibid. 280). In other words: for a problem that was transformed to and interpreted as an ethical problem, an "ethical solution" was found in the form of a national ethics committee. As the then head of state, President Mitterrand, said in his inaugural speech, the purpose of the CCNE was "not to impede the development of research or to impress norms on society, and especially on the society of practitioners and the learned, who you are" (Mitterrand 1987: 87; transl. SK), and in this way, its remit was similar to that of the proposed reflection group. Scientific self-government was modified into more open expert deliberation, without, however, questioning the legitimacy of research or decision-making.

"BIO"-GOVERNING THROUGH ETHICAL SPEECH: THE CCNE'S "OWN RULES OF LIVING"

Since its establishment in 1983, "ethical" expert deliberation in form of the CCNE seems to be characterized by not questioning the legitimacy of technological development. So, what is negotiated within the ethics frame and what is excluded? And, what does "ethics" mean with reference to the CCNE?

In its more than twenty-five-year existence, the CCNE has published more than one hundred opinions and recommendations on "ethical issues" in biotechnology and biomedicine. When I asked the members of the CCNE what they meant by the term ethics, the interview partners gave different and often vague answers. They explained, "Inasmuch as the concept of ethics pertains to the ethics committee, I think few people give much thought to the word." Another one said, "Morality, that's gray hair, the old generation, reactionaries who want to prescribe for us the things that they consider good. Ethics means: I make my own rules of living, independently." Or, "That is ethics for me: to turn to the public and communicate elements for reflection"; "… ethical reflection,… must always be measureed—…, nobody here asserts a claim to truth …." And, "My concept of ethics is that these instances make statements or recommendations, but not norms." Thus, while there is no common definition of ethics within the CCNE, interview partners agreed that "ethics"—in contradistinction to morality—is precisely an individual matter. For this individual matter, the committee communicates elements of reflection and stimulates debate, without a claim to norms or truth—and, as Mitterrand had already said in his inaugural speech in the year 1983 "neither for society nor for scientists" (ibid. 87).

Looking at the composition of the CCNE and its thirty-nine members, it is less a specific professional competence through which a person is qualified as a member of the CCNE than a certain attitude. The competency that a member must have is a capability for reasonable communication. In this way, according to two interviewed members of the French CCNE, the committee can be understood mainly as a national "pre-reflection committee" that provides a public model of reasonable conflict resolution and accommodation. For this mode of accommodation, it is important to maintain a moderate attitude. As one interviewed member put it with reference to the CCNE, "... ethical reflection ... must always be measured ...." Rather than making a "claim to truth," which would imply the falsity of opposing positions, players are committed to moderate accommodation of coexistent positions (see Memmi 1996). Those who take up an essential normative position lack the decisive competence of a "good" member: the ideal member is reflective, moderate, and has the flexible capability to see all positions and issues as discussable. The open and flexible attitude corresponds to the open and flexible, temporalized character of the recommendations that emerge from these discussions. An interviewee explained:

One must say that we do not see our position statements as the truth. If you like, our position statements are precarious, because we discuss at a specific point in time a state of knowledge that is evolving, and a moment of social acceptability that is also evolutionary. Our position statements are thus precarious and reversible. Perhaps they will no longer be warranted in 2007.

Participation in ethics discourses requires accepting that the outcomes are "evolutionary, reversible, and precarious." The public "ethical" discussion of these "precarious" and "reversible" statements or recommendations takes place in the form of annual public events, the *Journées annuelles d'éthique*. As a member of the CCNE explained in an interview, a particularly appreciated target group here are school students, because: "In this way naïve questions, lay questions can be posed, which provoke the ethics council to reflect. These days are an asset to the CCNE ...." According to a further interviewee the young people are seen as future citizens who are asked to cultivate "ethical" reflection and give their own presentations on "ethical" themes. The process is considered successful when the students understand that ethics means "examining the frame of reference" and that in "ethics" one can never arrive at definitive answers.[9] Didier Sicard, former president of the CCNE, supports this evaluation by proposing that the CCNE should be called "the national committee for ethical uncertainty" (Sicard 2001: 15; transl. SK). It is therefore not simply a matter of communicating scientific knowledge or ethical positions, but rather one of stimulating participants to deliberate, discuss, balance arguments, and form their individual temporarily valid opinions. Further, the "naïveté" of the young people is considered as being a specific resource for the members of the committee, as they provide ideas and views that can help to further enhance and stimulate future debates. At the same time, they function as "multipliers" who spread the art of ethical reflection among their families, as an interviewee said.

In addition, these public discourses have an educational dimension. They offer an opportunity for participants to practice the proper style of ethical reflection—"proper" referring not to the quality of substantive judgments, but to the style of thinking and speaking about the issues. This style excludes a certain kind of speaker position. In the context of biotechnological issues, one overlooked objection by a student at the *Journées annuelles* of the CCNE was that on the grounds of over-production, the issue was not the further technical development of genetically manipulated plants, but rather above all a question of distribution. In contrast, the reaction of a member of the CCNE to a participant's statement that did not question scientific progress was, "You have understood the difficulties and the problematization."[10] So, the "proper ethical speech" is not to have a position but to employ the proper mode of reflection. And that means not questioning scientific progress. The ignored contribution of a participant at the *Journées annuelles d'éthique* shows that discussions about scientific development itself are not integrated into the ethical debate on biotechnological issues. It seems that "ethics" in the sense of the CCNE in biotechnological discourse avoids substantive answers. It is more a style of managing thinking and reflecting in the "proper" way: individually, perpetually, measured. The characteristic of "ethics" is the no-go of questioning scientific development or arguing in an antagonistic way. Are these characteristics of "ethics" to be found in nanotechnological discourses as well?

---

9   *Journées annuelles d'éthique* (16–17 Nov 2004), Université Paris V René Descartes, Paris. SK attended the conference.

10 Ibid.

"ETHICS" IN NANOTECHNOLOGICAL DISCOURSE: "SCIENCE LEAPS AHEAD"?!

The language of ethics in biotechnological discourses has emerged in the context of questioning versus stabilizing scientific self-government and in the context of the anticipation of criticism. So, are there analogous characteristics in the discourse on nanotechnology?

In nanotechnological discourses, whose origins date back to the year 1959,[11] an explicit framing in the language of ethics appeared only much later. Until the beginning of the new millennium, the discourses on nanotechnology remained mainly within scientific circles and were concentrated on a small number of players and events, for the most part in the US. The discourses were characterized by a conflict over what is to be understood by nanotechnology (Berube/Shipman 2004; Wullweber 2008). Therefore, it was also an implicit conflict about what the ethical issues are, but a perceivable framing in terms of ethics appeared only some years later. Meanwhile, the most frequently applied definition of nanotechnology is the following: "Nanotechnology is everything that occupies the scale of the nanometer" (Glimell/Fogelberg 2003: 19; Wullweber 2008: 29).

While in the US, nanotechnologies were discussed as early as in the 1990s, in Europe the debate started at the beginning of the new millennium and is framed in a mixture of risk and ethics. The key event was a public intervention by Prince Charles in July 2003, where he warned about the possible dangers of nanotechnologies and especially of the so-called gray goo effect[12] (Daily Mail 2003). Prince Charles' intervention had already

---

11 In 1959, physicist Richard Feynmann gave the lecture There's plenty of Room at the Bottom at the California Institute of Technology (Feynmann 1959). Although he did not mention the term nanotechnology, he is regarded as the "father of nanotechnology," as he formulated a paradigm shift of miniaturization. His idea was not only to miniaturize things, but to construct them with particles (Schaper-Rinkel 2006: 473).

12 Gray Goo is the vision of destruction of life that could result from the accidental and uncontrollable spread of so called self-replicating nanobots (a kind of robot). The term was coined by K. Eric Drexler in his book Engines of Creation in the mid-1980s (Drexler 1987). Bill Joy took Drexler's apocalyptic vision of nanotechnology to a wider public (Joy 2000b).

been preceded by calls for abandonment of and a moratorium for the development and applications of nanotechnology, through which it reached a wider public: in 2000, the article Why the Future doesn't need Us was published by US scientist Bill Joy[13] in the IT magazine Wired (Joy 2000b) as well as in the French daily newspaper *Le Monde* (Joy 2000a). Joy pointed out the impacts of new technologies such as genetics, nanotechnology, and robotics and called for their renunciation: in the face of uncertain and limited knowledge about technological progress and the far-ranging potentials of nanotechnology, there would be risks that could be avoided only by doing without the development and application of such technologies. The problematization by the critical scientific association ETC Group, an international NGO, pronounced at the World Summit on Sustainable Development in Johannesburg in 2002 is similar (Mnyusiwalla/Daar/Singer 2003). The group calls for a moratorium on the diffusion of nanomaterials due to the "incalculable risks" (ETC Group 2003: 72). Prince Charles' intervention, publications by international NGOs, such as the ETC Group, and the environmental organization Greenpeace initiated a public debate in France (Arnall 2003; ETC Group 2003; Vinck/Gallice/Jouvenet/Zarama 2009). At the same time, the first publications in the field of social sciences and bioethics appeared to analyze the call for a moratorium and the advancing research and development as a schism: "As the science leaps ahead, the ethics lags behind" (Mnyusiwalla/Daar/Singer 2003: R9f.). It is problematized as a development similar to the case of genetically modified organisms (GMO). The solution is seen in "research into the ethical, legal, and social implications of NT"[14] (Baumgartner 2004; Mnyusiwalla/Daar/Singer 2003; R1; Roco 2003). The recommendation of "more ethics" but also the evaluation of "opportunities and risks" was to be found at the informal meeting International Dialogue on Responsible Research and Development of Nanotechnology in 2004. The dialogue took place in Alexandria, Virginia, upon invitation of the US National Nanotechnology Initiative[15] (Tomellini 2004). At this multidisciplinary expert meeting, in which experts from twenty-five countries, including France, participated, "socioeconomic and

---

13 Joy is Chief Scientist of the computer and software company Sun Microsystems.
14 NT: Nanotechnology.
15 The National Nanotechnology Initiative is a federal nanoscale science, engineering, technology research, and development program.

ethical implications" of nanotechnologies were discussed in particular. The participants "agreed to continue the process and to explore ways of encouraging broader social dialogue" (ibid. 2004). France was represented by the *Conseil général des technologies et de l'information*, a governmental institution (until 2009) that had a safeguarding function in the area of technologies, especially information technologies. In 2004, it published the report "Nanotechnologies: Ethics and Industrial Perspectives" (Dupuy/Roure 2004; transl. SK). The aim of the report was to prepare the principal axes of evaluation of French public policies with regard to nanotechnology, especially concerning the social and ethical implications (ibid.). As for "ethics," the report states specifically: "There must be an ethics that is infinitely more exigent than the one which is slowly being established today for containing the rhythm and the possible developments in biotechnologies" (ibid. 27; transl. SK). Furthermore, the report encourages institutions and bodies to explore the "risks" and "ethics" of nanotechnology and presents the CCNE as a positive model. The CCNE had already established a working group on nanotechnology in 2004 (ibid. 67). "Ethics" as conflict prevention can be found in further publications in ensuing years: a report by the *Centre d'analyse stratégique*, the governmental "Center for Strategic Analysis" (transl. SK), on "Nanotechnologies: Anticipating dealing with Risks" stated "ethical and social fears" (Centre d'analyse stratégique 2006: 3; transl. SK). These "fears" could: "... stoke an attitude of mistrust of science that is dangerous in its evolution in a context marked by the controversies over GMO ..." (ibid. transl. SK). Likewise, a report by the *Office parlementaire d'évaluation des choix scientifiques et technologiques* (Parliamentary Office for the Evaluation of Scientific and Technological Choices, OPECST) declared that, in the context of nanotechnologies, a situation of trust does not exist among the public, and that the "GMO syndrome" was to be avoided in advance (OPECST 2006: 6; transl. SK). On the governmental level, a development has been problematized not in analogy to the discourse about nuclear technology, but to the one on genetic engineering. Apart from the conflicts about genetic engineering in the 1970s, which remained confined to scientific circles of research institutes, controversies about this technology have been increasing since the 1990s in France, mainly in the agricultural field. Additional background for this problematization are the controversies on the regional level in Grenoble around the research centre *Minatec*[16] (see Vinck/Gallice/Jouvenet/Zarama 2009). A group of activists called *Pièces et main d'oeuvre* (PMO) has been criticizing the research projects in the region of Grenoble since 2002. They have organized demonstrations, disturbed public meetings, and held alternative discussions about the dangers of nanotechnology (Laurent 2007: 345). As to PMO's critique, a similar techno-skeptical attitude is obvious not only in the controversies about genetic engineering (from thirty years ago), but also as a critique of scientific decision-making (ibid. 348f): not only are the technological dangers for society made a topic of discussion, but also expert domination or capitalist interests in decision-making (Cette Semaine 2004; Rebellyon 2010). In contrast to the ethical framing of biotechnological issues, however, the ethical framing in nanotechnological discourse is disputed. Critics emphasize, "We smell that the 'ethical' flatteries ... are nothing more than clean camouflages of *faits accomplis*" (Simples Citoyens 2003: 17; transl. SK). While on the governmental level it is stated: "In any case, the issues are ethical, commercial, and issues of public health" (OPECST 2006: 46; transl. SK), PMO counters: "We offer you—cost-free and voluntarily—a 'minimal introduction to nanotechnologies' that describes our critique—not technical critique, but political, philosophical, social, and ecological" (Pièces et Main d'Oeuvre 2006; transl. SK). While PMO's critique is not framed in terms of ethics, similar to the controversies in biotechnology in the 1970s, conflicts in the context of nanotechnology and their expansion in terms of the GMO controversies are indeed anticipated by governmental institutions and framed in the language of ethics. Governmental institutions argue that there *are* "ethical and social fears" or "emotions" that require an effective response by means of a "rational" public debate (OPECST 2006: 126), organized in citizen conferences to discuss "ethical considerations" or by ethics committees. These "ethical fears" and "emotions" are situated on the side of society and become something that

---

16 The research centre *Minatec* was founded as early as 1998 by the public establishment *Commissariat à l'énergie atomique et aux énergies alternatives* (Callon/Dianoux/Fourniau/Gilbert et al 2005: 12). The agreement that constituted *Minatec* was signed in 2002 and its opening ceremony was held in 2006 (Laurent 2007: 345).

has to be "cured" via the involvement of citizens in the "proper" rational debate. Furthermore, it is obvious that it is contested whether nanotechnological issues are ethical or political issues. But it seems that the framing of nanotechnological issues as issues of health and ethics has become accepted, mainly at the governmental level. Meanwhile, the OPECST (ibid.), COMETS, the ethics committee of the National Centre of Scientific Research (COMETS 2006), a citizen conference on the regional level (Île de France 2006), and the CCNE have been engaged with "ethical issues" of nanotechnology (CCNE 2007). The same holds true for the public debates held in seventeen French cities organized by the National Commission of Public Debate taking into account "legitimate ethical questions" (Commission nationale du débat public 2009: 5; transl. SK).[17] So, it can be stated that there is a stimulation of public "ethical" debate and a proliferation of ethical framing.

"NANO"-GOVERNING THROUGH ETHICAL SPEECH: IS EVERYTHING IN GOOD HEALTH?

The language of ethics in nanotechnological discourse appears similar to that used in the discourses on biotechnology in the 1970s for rejecting techno-skeptical viewpoints and actions. But, do the characteristics of the CCNE's ethical framing of biotechnological issues—the concentration on the management of one's own health and the indisputability of scientific development—also apply to nanotechnological issues? Has the ethical framing changed over time and with respect to nanotechnology?

In 2007, the CCNE published its first opinion on nanotechnology titled Ethical Issues raised by Nanosciences, Nanotechnologies, and Health (CCNE 2007). Not only the title but also the following quotation show that the CCNE inevitably frames "ethical" issues as health issues, whether they directly concern the human body or not: "Ethics covers here a complex multidisciplinary array of issues ranging from the possible effects on health of nanoparticles used for non medical purposes through to the benefits and risks of nanomedicine and the human sciences" (ibid. 7). "Health" as well

---

17 For an overview of further public debates on nanotechnology in France (and Europe), see Papilloud 2010.

as "ethics" are framed as individual matters. Aside from public information about nanotechnological development, "[i]ndustrialists must be required to provide information and clear specific labelling of products containing nanoparticles so that consumers can refuse to use them if they so wish" (ibid. 15). In the CCNE's opinion, "ethics" is not a question of economic development, which is not discussed, but a stimulus to individual decision-making regarding one's own health. Furthermore, it is not only an individual matter for consumers but also for future scientists and medical practitioners in the field of nanotechnology, who are called upon to write a summary about their ethical reflection in their doctoral theses (ibid. 13). And it is recommended that scientists as well as engineers and economic decision-makers are trained in "ethics" (ibid. 12f).

In the context of biotechnological issues, members of the CCNE characterized the kind of ethical reflection as "evolutionary, reversible, and precarious." This kind of reflection has not changed over time. One interview partner stated: "It is an endless questioning of what we see as values" and "the principle of ethical reflection does not mean to say what is good or bad." In other words, there is only one principle for "ethical" deliberation for both bio- and nanotechnological issues: the principle of endless reflection. In the context of biotechnological issue, this endless reflection does not include the questioning of technological development. Similarly, in the context of nanotechnological issues, a member of the CCNE stated: "The ethical reflection that we conduct especially within the CCNE isn't aimed at all at slowing down scientific progress, but to call for more science, more research ..." (OPECST 2006: 52; transl. SK). Similar characteristics can be found in the ethical framing of both bio- and nanotechnological issues: the framing of the issues as health and individual issues, the temporalized or endless character of reflection, and the indisputability of ongoing research and development. By way of these analogies it seems that "ethics" is flexible and interchangeable with other policy issues, such as nanotechnology.

CONCLUSIONS

In both biotechnological and nanotechnological discourses, the language of ethics has emerged in the context of questioning versus stabilizing scientific self-government and in the context of the anticipation and transformation or "ethicization" of the political criticism of scientific decision-making. The institutionalization of "ethics" in the form of the French National Consultative Ethics Committee on Health and Life Sciences, established in 1983, is the result of opposing imperatives: On the one hand there was the problem of a certain social order—scientific self-government had become a problem. It was no longer taken as self-evident but recognized as a form of government that required justification and modification. On the other hand, scientific development was not to be impeded. The solution to this problem of squaring the circle is institutionalized processualization: permanent reflection and dialogue on the part of a national ethics committee (Braun/Herrmann/Könninger/Moore 2008: 228). This permanent and "flexible" reflection is possible because neither norms, truth, the good, nor the bad are produced within the ethics frame. The latter would impede accommodation, for it would assert that opposing positions would be false. Concerning the CCNE, it seems that "ethics," both in bio- and nanotechnological discourses, implies the exclusion of certain speaker positions and arguments, such as those which include a more general interrogation of techno-scientific development and of scientific governance itself. As to the CCNE, it seems that the "magistère bioéthique" has been expanded to nanotechnological issues insofar as "nanoethics" focuses on individual decision-making referring to one's own health and insofar as "responsibility" is delegated to the individual. However the further question is how "ethics" is framed within other procedures, such as the public dialogues organized in France.

As to scientific governance and the CCNE, "ethics" provides a frame for the production and organization of discourse rather than a substantial normative orientation for action. Bio- and nanotechnological discourses share the characteristic: "Everything has to be possible, with one exception: Saying no" (Braun/Herrmann/Könninger/Moore 2009; transl. SK).

REFERENCES

Alias, François (1992): Le comité consultatif national d'éthique et l'institutionnalisation d'un débat public relatif à l'éthique biomédicale. Approche critique, Institut des sciences sociales Raymond Ledrut, Université Toulouse-Le Mirail, Microfiche: Toulouse.

Arnall, Alexander Huw (2003): Future technologies, today's choices: nanotechnology, artificial intelligence and robotics; a technical, political and institutional map of emerging technologies. A report for the Greenpeace Environmental Trust, 7/2003, London; available at http://www.greenpeace.org.uk/files/pdfs/migrated/MultimediaFiles/ Live/FullReport/5886.pdf (last accessed 8/20/2008).

Baumgartner, Peter (2004): "Ethische Aspekte nanotechnologischer Forschung und Entwicklung in der Medizin", in: Aus Politik und Zeitgeschichte B 23-24, pp. 39–46.

Berg, Paul/Baltimore, David/Boyer, Herbert W./Cohen, Stanley N. et al (1974): "Potential biohazards of recombinant DNA molecules", in: Science 185, p. 303.

Berube, David/Shipman, J.D. (2004): "Denialism: Drexler vs. Roco", in: Technology and Society Magazine IEEE 23, pp. 22–26; available at http://ieeexplore.ieee.org/stamp/stamp.jsp?tp=&arnumber=1371635&is number=29989 (last accessed 5/18/2009).

Braun, Kathrin/Herrmann, Svea Luise/Könninger, Sabine/Moore, Alfred (2008): "Die Sprache der Ethik und die Politik des richtigen Sprechens? Ethikregime in Deutschland, Frankreich und Großbritannien", in: Renate Mayntz/Friedhelm Neidhardt/Peter Weingart/Ulrich Wengenroth (eds), Wissensproduktion und Wissenstransfer. Wissen im Spannungsfeld von Wissenschaft, Politik und Öffentlichkeit, Bielefeld: transcript, pp. 221–242.

— (2009): "Bioethik in der Politik", in: Aus Politik und Zeitgeschichte. 8(19), pp. 40–46.

— (2010a): "Ethical reflection must always be measured", in: Science Technology & Human Values 35(6), pp. 839-864.

Braun, Kathrin/Moore, Alfred/Herrmann, Svea Luise/Könninger, Sabine (2010b): "Science governance and the politics of proper talk: governmental bioethics as a new technology of reflexive government", in: Economy and Society 39(4), pp. 510-533.

Callon, Michel/Dianoux, Laurent/Fourniau, Jean-Michel/Gilbert, Claude et al (2005): Democratie locale et maîtrise sociale des nanotechnologies. Les publics grenoblois peuvent-ils participer aux choix scientifiques et techniques? Rapport de la Mission pour La Métro. Rapport final, 22 septembre 2005, pp. 1-58; available at http://sciencescitoyennes.org/

IMG/pdf/NanoGrenoble_rapport_final_05_09_22.pdf (last accessed 10/12/2007).

CCNE (2007): Opinion N°96. Ethical issues raised by nanosciences, nanotechnologies and health, pp. 1–18; available at http://www.ccne-ethique.fr/docs/en/avis096.pdf (last accessed 6/3/2010).

Cette Semaine (2004): Grenoble, occupation d'une grue du chantier Minatec; available at http://cettesemaine.free.fr/article.php3?id_article=31 (last accessed 12/10/2007).

COMETS (2006): Avis. Enjeux Ethiques. Des Nanosciences et nanotechnologies. CNRS, rendu le 12 octobre 2006, pp. 1-25; available at http://www.cnrs.fr/fr/presentation/ethique/comets/index.htm (last accessed 1/12/2007).

Commission nationale du débat public (2009): Débat public sur les options générales en matière de développement et de régulation des nanotechnologies. Dossier de presse, 15 octobre 2009 au 24 février 2010, pp. 1-13; available at http://www.debatpublic-nano.org/presse/dossier_presse.html?id_document=38 (last accessed 9/30/2009).

Daily Mail (2003): "Stay out of politics Charles, says Lord Sainsbury (the unelected billionaire Minister and major Labour donor)", in: Daily Mail, 6/17/2003; available at http://www.agbioworld.org/biotech-info/articles/biotech-art/princecharles.html (last accessed 5/21/2006).

Drexler, K. Eric (1987): Engines of creation, New York: Anchor Press.

Dupuy, Jean-Pierre/Roure, Françoise (2004): Les Nanotechnologies: Éthique et prospectice industrielle. Conseil Général des Mines; Conseil Général des Technologies de l'Information, pp. 1–73; available at http://admi.net/cgi-bin/wiki?Nanotechnologies (last accessed 7/21/2008).

ETC Group (2003): The big down. From genomes to atoms, pp. 1-84; available at http://www.etcgroup.org/en/materials/publications.html?pub_id=171 (last accessed 3/28/2007).

Evans, John H. (2002): Playing God: human genetic engineering and the rationalization of the public bioethical debate, Chicago: University of Chicago press.

Feynmann, Richard P. (1959): Plenty of room at the bottom; available at http://www.its.caltech.edu/~feynman/plenty.html (last accessed 8/4/2008).

Foucault, Michel (1991): "Governmentality", in: Graham Burchell/Colin Gordon/Peter Miller (eds), The Foucault effect: studies in governmentality, London: Harvester Wheatsheaf, pp. 87–194.

Galpérine, Charles (1976): Biologie et devenir de l'homme: actes du colloque mondial, 18-24 septembre 1974, Paris: McGraw Hill.

Glimell, Hans/Fogelberg, Hans (2003): "Molecular matters: in search of the real stuff", in: Hans Glimell/Hans Fogelberg (eds), Bringing visibility to the invisible: towards a social understanding of nanotechnology, in: STS Research Reports 6, Göteborg University, pp. 4–28.

Gros, François/Jacob, François/Royer, Pierre (1979): Sciences de la vie et société. Rapport présenté à M. le Président de la République, Paris: La documentation française.

Herrmann, Svea/Könninger, Sabine (2008): ""... but you cannot influence the direction of your thinking": guiding self-government in bioethics policy discourse", in: Elizabeth Mitchell Armstrong/Barbara Katz Rothman/Rebecca Tiger (eds), Bioethical Issues, Sociological Perspectives (=Advances in Medical Sociology, 9), Amsterdam: Elsevier JAI, pp. 205-223.

Herrmann, Svea Luise (2009): Policy debates on reprogenetics. The problematisation of new research in Great Britain and Germany, Frankfurt a. M.: Campus.

Île de France (2006): La conférence de citoyens sur les nanotechnologies: explorons les enjeux de l'infiniment petit. Conférence de presse du 10 octobre 2006, pp. 1–3; available at http://espaceprojets.iledefrance.fr/jahia/webdav/site/projets/users/JLACHKAR/public/communiqu%C3%A9%20du%2010-10-06.pdf (last accessed 11/22/2006).

Irwin, Alan (2006): "The politics of talk: coming to terms with 'new' scientific governance", in: Social Studies of Science 36, pp. 299–320.

Jömann, Norbert/Ach, Johann S. (2006): "Ethical implications of nanobiotechnology—a state-of-the-art survey of ethical issues related to nanobiotechnology", in: Johann S. Ach/Ludwig Siep, Nano-bio-ethics. Ethical dimensions of nanobiotechnology, Berlin: Lit, pp. 13–62.

Joy, Bill (2000a): "Restructurer le genre humain", in: Le Monde, 7/5/2000.

— (2000b): "Why the future doesn't need us", in: Wired 12; available at http://www.wired.com/wired/archive/8.04/joy_pr.html (last accessed 7/30/2008).

Kelly, Susan E. (2003): "Public bioethics and publics: consensus, boundaries, and participation in biomedical science policy", in: Science, Technology & Human Values 28, pp. 339–364; available at http://sth.sagepub.com/cgi/reprint/28/3/339 (last accessed 8/28/2008).

Könninger, Sabine (2009): 'From bioethics to nanoethics?' Development, institutionalisation and framing of ethics policy in France. Paper presented at the 4th International Conference in Interpretive Policy Analysis: Discourse and Power in Critical Policy Studies, 25-27 Jun 2009. Methodological Workshop, University of Kassel.

— (2010): "From bio to nano? Governing through ethical speech in France", in: Ulrich Fiedeler/Christopher Coenen/Sarah R. Davies/Arianna Ferrari (eds), Understanding nanotechnology: philosophy, policy and publics, Heidelberg: AKA, pp. 121-132.

Krauss, Gerhard (1996): Forschung im unitaristischen Staat. Abhängigkeit und Autonomie der staatlich finanzierten Forschung in Frankreich. Frankfurt a. M.: Campus.

Krimsky, Sheldon (1982): Genetic alchemy: the social history of the recombinant DNA controversy, Cambridge: MIT Press.

Laurent, Brice (2007): "Diverging convergences", in: Innovation: The European Journal of Social Science Research 20, pp. 343–357, available at http://cns.asu.edu/cns-library/documents/Laurent_DivergingCon vergences_07.pdf (last accessed 11/11/2008).

Levidow, Les/Carr, Susan (1997): "How biotechnology regulation sets a risk/ethics boundary", in: Agriculture and Human Values 14, pp. 29–43.

Memmi, Dominique (1996): Les gardiens du corps? Dix ans de magistère bioéthique, Paris: Editions de l'Ecole des hautes études en sciences sociales.

— (2003a): Faire vivre et laisser mourir. Le gouvernement contemporain de la naissance et de la mort, Paris: Editions de l'Ecole des hautes études en sciences sociales.

— (2003b): "Governing through speech. The new state administration of bodies", in: Social Research 70, pp. 645–658.

— (2005): La "bio-politique déléguée": L'institution serait-elle soluble dans le retour du "sujet"? Paper presented at the Colloque international. Le politique vu avec Foucault, 7-8 Jan 2005, Paris: IEP and CIR.

Mendel, Agata (1980): Les manipulations génétique, Paris: Le Seuil.

Mitterrand, François (1987): "Allocution prononcée par M. François Mitterrand, Président de la République française, à l'occasion de la mise en place du Comité consultatif national d'éthique pour les sciences de la vie et de la santé. Vendredi 2 décembre 1983", in: Comités d'éthique à travers du monde. Recherches en cours 1986, pp. 85–88.

Mnyusiwalla, Anisa/Daar, Abdallah S./Singer, Peter A. (2003): "'Mind the gap': science and ethics in nanotechnology", in: Nanotechnology 14, pp. R9-R13; available at http://stacks.iop.org/Nano/14/R9 (last accessed 4/16/2008).

Mouvement de la responsabilité scientifique (2005): Qu'est ce que le M.U.R.S.?; available at http://www.murs-france.asso.fr/Presentation/C_present.html (last accessed 6/5/2005).

Namur, Dominique (2006): Nanotechnologies: Anticiper pour gérer les risques, in: Centre d'analyse stratégique, La note de veille, 27(25 septembre 2006); available at http://www.strategie.gouv.fr/IMG/pdf/noteveille27.pdf (last accessed 5/11/2008).

OPECST (2006): Les Nanotechnologies: Risques potentiels, enjeux éthiques, Compte rendue de l'audition publique du 7 novembre. Paris, pp. 1–137; available at http://www.assemblee-nationale.fr/12/pdf/rap-off/i3658.pdf (last accessed 7/7/2008).

Papilloud, Christian (2010): Gouverner l'infiniment petit. Les nanotechnologies à Grenoble et Hambourg, Paris: L'Harmattan.

Pièces et Main d'Oeuvre (2006): Pièces et Main d'Oeuvre écrit aux députés; available at http://www.piecesetmaindoeuvre.com/spip.php?page=resume&id_article=91 (last accessed 4/27/2009).

Rebellyon (2010): Nano-débats pour maxi-arnaque; available at http://rebellyon.info/Nano-debats-pour-maxi-arnaque.html (last accessed 11/16/2010).

Rein, Martin/Schön, Donald (1993): "Reframing policy discourse", in: Frank Fischer/John Forrester (eds), The argumentative turn in policy analysis and planning, Durham: Duke University Press, pp. 145–166.

Roco, M.C. (2003): "Broader societal issues of nanotechnology", in: Journal of Nanoparticle Research 5, pp. 181–189.

Schaper-Rinkel, Petra (2006): "Governance von Zukunftsversprechen: Zur politischen Ökonomie der Nanotechnologie", in: PROKLA, Zeitschrift für kritische Sozialwissenschaft 135(36), pp. 471–426; available at http://www.prokla.de/Volltexte/volltextframeset.htm (last accessed 5/5/ 2007).

Sicard, Didier (2001): "Erfahrungsberichte. Ethikräte in Frankreich und der Europäischen Union", in: Berliner Dialog zu Biomedizin, pp. 10–15; available at http://www.fes-landesbuero-berlin.de/doku/01_02.pdf (last accessed 3/12/2004).

Simples Citoyens (2003): Nanotechnologies/Maxiservitude. Des contributions grenobloises à l'automatisation du cheptel humain; available at http://www.piecesetmaindoeuvre.com/IMG/pdf/Nanotechnologies-maxi servitude.pdf (last accessed 7/22/2006).

Tomellini, Renzo (2004): International dialogue on responsible research and development of nanotechnology. 17-18 Jun 2004, Alexandria, VA; available at ftp://ftp.cordis.europa.eu/pub/nanotechnology/docs/alex andria062004.pdf (last accessed 6/9/2010).

Touraine, Alain (1982): Die antinukleare Prophetie. Zukunftsentwürfe einer sozialen Bewegung. Frankfurt a. M.: Campus.

Vinck, Dominique/Gallice, Perrine/Jouvenet, Morgan/Zarama, Gloria (2009): Dynamique technologique controversée et débat démocratique: le cas des micro- et nanotechnologies; available at http://halshs. archives-ouvertes.fr/docs/00/36/00/74/PDF/060718_ChapVinck_ GOUJON_V1.pdf (last accessed 2/21/2010).

Wullweber, Joscha (2008): "Nanotechnology – an empty signifier à venir? A delineation of a techno-socio-economical innovation strategy", in: Science, Technology & Innovation Studies 4, pp. 27–45.

New biopolitics? The articulation of demographic aims and gender policies in international population programs

SUSANNE SCHULTZ

In recent years, a number of researchers in governmentality studies[1] have claimed to trace the emergence of a new global regime of biopolitics (Heath/Rapp/Taussig 2004; Lemke 2000; 2004; Rabinow/Rose 2003; Rose 2001; Rose/Novas 2002). This new regime, they posit, is no longer based on the management of the population as a whole, and its novelty lies in the development of new forms of "biological citizenship." They argue that it has become increasingly inadequate to frame current biopolitics in terms of biological determinism and reductionism, of state-led population policies, or of eugenics and racism.[2]

In this paper, I will argue that these assumptions turn out to be misleading if we look at one important field of international biopolitics, namely

---

1 Regarding the governmentality concept, see Foucault 2004; for an introduction to governmentality studies, see Burchell/Gordon/Miller 1993 and Bröckling/Krasmann/Lemke 2000.
2 There are differences, though, as to what extent governmentality scholars question older forms of critique: While Nikolas Rose questions the "older" approaches more fundamentally, Thomas Lemke integrates them but emphasizes that they are no longer sufficient (2000).

international population policies directed at reducing world population growth. I will argue that we can understand current biopolitics better if we start from a more complex analysis of articulation between totalizing demographic and individualizing medicalizing rationalities. Referring to the concept of articulation, as elaborated by Ernesto Laclau and Chantal Mouffe (1991), I understand articulation as a process in which discursive elements change their meaning when they are related and linked to one another.[3] In the case at hand, I will show that the success story of new individualizing concepts, like reproductive health and rights, as they have emerged on the population agenda since the United Nations' International Conference on Population and Development in Cairo in 1994, can only be fully understood if we analyze these concepts as articulated with state-led demographic strategies.

In the following, I will first argue that current governmentality studies oftentimes refer to the Foucauldian concept of biopolitics in a one-sided way. In the second part of the paper, I will analyze the articulation of demographic aims and gender policies in international population programs and interpret them as an articulation of selective, racist forms of population management and the promotion of individual responsibilities in "reproductive risk" management.

THEORETICAL ASSUMPTIONS ABOUT NEW BIOPOLITICS

The empirical focus of current governmentality studies on new biopolitics is primarily on new developments in biomedical arenas, especially on genetic, genomic, and reproductive technologies and related social and cultural changes in dealing with reproduction, health, and corporality in the advanced liberal societies of the West. Nevertheless, the explanatory claim of these works exceeds these thematic areas by far. Nikolas Rose and his co-authors' theses can serve as a case in point of how these studies criticize older approaches to biopolitics as inadequate (Rabinow/Rose 2003; Rose

---

3   That does not mean that I fully agree with all aspects of their social theory project. For instance, I object to extending the field of hegemonic discursive articulation to the social per se, a project which tends towards idealistic politicism (see Jessop 1990: 289).

2001; Rose/Novas 2002).[4] According to Rose and this collaborators, present biopolitics can no longer be understood as the national management of a constructed, uniform entity, be it a people, a biological race, or a homogeneous population (Rabinow/Rose 2003: 25, 33; Rose 2001: 5; Rose/Novas 2002: 8). Instead, we are dealing with a dispositif of genetic or body policies that establishes a host of functional and probabilistic differentiations regarding either health or the body, thus creating knowledge that serves as the basis for individuals to manage and enhance their bodies in an active way. "The norm of individual health replaced that of the quality of the population". (Rose 2001: 13; see ibid: 7; Rabinow/Rose 2003: 26; Rose/Novas 2002: 5) The state is becoming less important in this biopolitical regime and is being replaced with or at least supplemented by both global and decentralized networks and by economic rationalities connected to new biotechnologies (Rabinow/Rose 2003: 15f, 35; Rose 2001: 5f.).[5] In Rose's words: "Biopolitics becomes bioeconomics". (Rose 2001: 15)

Rose stresses that current biopolitics–referring to the poles of biopolitics in Foucault's analysis–function on a biopolitical micro-level, namely the individualized reference to the body and health behavior rather than on the macro-level, that is, the regulation of populations (Rose 2001: 12; see Rabinow/Rose 2003: 15). This micro-level, according to Rose, is the dynamic and crucial basis for a new biopolitics because now individual (and also collective) subjects are activated and mobilized through self-responsibility for their bodies and health. Hence, Rose views the emergence of new self-technologies and new subjectivities framed in terms such as empowerment, autonomy, and informed consent as paradigmatic for this new form of biopolitics. In this context, Rose and his co-authors concede that the new subjectivities are characterized by an increasing biologization of individual and collective identity formation; they speak of an emerging

---

4 Although Rose shields his theses by making a variety of concessions to "older" biopolitical constellations that still exist today, I think, criticism of the main thrust of his arguments is justified.

5 In Rose and Novas' view, the population as an entity is, if at all, mostly relevant to the state as an economic resource, for instance, as a "genomic goldmine," as genetic biodiversity that provides "biovalue" through biobanks or pharmacogenomics, through products and patents, thus becoming a factor in the international struggle for competitiveness (Rose/Novas 2003: 29-31).

"biosociality" (Rabinow/Rose 2003: 36; Rose 2001: 18). However, Rose et al argue that biological ascription is not appropriately understood in terms of a passively accepted fate and determinism but rather as a sphere holding a wide range of opportunities for shaping one's life and for "self-enhancement" and also providing scope for the sort of "biological citizenship" (Rose/Novas 2002) emerging today.

Rose and Rabinow refer to the Foucauldian concept of biopolitics as an analytical tool inasmuch as it aims to combine the analysis of knowledge production, power relations, and forms of subjectivization in the "politics of life." However, they believe that his analysis concerning the micro- and macro-dimension of biopolitics, respectively the relation between them, is out-dated when it comes to contemporary biopolitics (Rabinow/Rose 2003: 14). In my view, this research strategy tends to neglect the productive tension in Foucault's concept of biopolitics between liberal governmentality and individualized self-technologies on the one hand, and biopolitical government, macro-political state-led regulation of populations and enduring forms of racism and biopolitical selection, on the other. In order to deal with the specific tension between liberal, individualized forms of conduct on the one hand, and ongoing racism and the selective management of the population as a whole, on the other–a tension that is crucial to the analyses of Foucault–I argue that we have to examine the "macro" side of biopolitics and not lose sight of it. In my view, we also need to understand the macro-political rationalities of heteronomy in order to understand present forms of self-governance. After all, the question of how constellations of dominance influence, although not determine, the emergence and exercise of self-technologies is the key question of the governmentality concept as such (Burchell 1993). Thus, not only the economic dimensions of "biovalue"–a concept developed by Catherine Waldby, which plays an important role for Rose–but also state-led population management continues to have an impact today (Rose 2001: 15; see Waldby 2000).

Related to the tension between macro- and micro-biopolitics is another issue: the tension between governmentality and racism in liberalism. Governmentality scholars tend to stress the individualizing and activating dimension of liberalism while rejecting its selective, racist dimension, a dimension that had been crucial to Foucault's concept of biopolitics (Foucault 1983: 166; see Gutiérrez Rodríguez 2003). Foucault emphasizes that it was through this racist dimension of biopolitics that it remained possible in liberalism to intervene into the structure of the population and to maintain the death-function in the economy of biopower despite the liberal accentuation of individual rights and freedom (Foucault 2001: 300-302; 2003: 1020). The racism of modern biopolitics, he argues, consists of justifying selective segregation within the population body by referring to an alleged optimization of life in general (Foucault 1983: 163; 2001: 302). In this understanding of racism, racism cannot be reduced to eugenics or genetic discrimination, as governmentality studies on biopolitics often, at least implicitly, suggest with their focus on racism based on the idea of a "biological substrate" (Rabinow/Rose 2003: 18; see Rose 2001: 3).[6] I hold that the neo-Malthusian logic which emphasizes the carrying capacity of the planet and questions the right to existence of the socially and economically excluded populations for the sake of saving the life of all, is still an important underlying rationale of racist global biopolitics that should not be neglected.

INTERNATIONAL POPULATION POLICIES AS AN ANACHRONISTIC FIELD OF RESEARCH

One of the problems with the idea of "new biopolitics," in my view, is that it is based on a focus mainly on new biotechnologies within the context of Western high-tech capitalism, thereby presuming, although not explicitly, certain hierarchies of research topics. General hypotheses about today's biopolitics are often derived from viewing a specific field of research, especially innovations within biomedicine, as the most advanced or central feature of current biopolitics, without reflecting on the limits of that particular field of research.

In contrast to the current concept of biopolitics focussing on new biotechnologies, critical social theory, in the heydays of internationalist movements from the late 1960s to the early 1990s, observed and analyzed international population policies as central to developing an internationalist anti-imperialist, anti-racist, and/or feminist critique (see Bradish/Feyerabend/Winkler 1989; Mass 1976). However, since the United Nations' In-

---

6   Rabinow and Rose cite this Foucauldian conceptualization of racism, but they do not consider it when classifying neo-Malthusian politics as non-eugenic and in this sense non-racist (see Rabinow/Rose 2003: 9, 25).

ternational Conference on Population and Development in Cairo (ICPD) in 1994, which established a reform agenda for international population policies, the international social science scene has largely ignored the topic as supposedly "anachronistic."[7] At the same time, population programs have remained an expanding sector of international development policies after 1994 (UNFPA 2004a) and a core paradigm of international health programs. From 1999 to 2004, population policy funding (excluding HIV/AIDS programs) accounted for 18 percent of overall health aid compared to 14 percent for basic healthcare and 7 percent for basic health infrastructure (OECD 2010).

In one dimension of the post-Cairo policies, the contemporary diagnoses by governmentality studies regarding new biopolitics also hold true for post-Cairo population programs: they are all characterized by a transformation of "programmatic subjectivities." By stressing "programmatic," I intend to point out that I will confine my analysis to the study of the struggles over how subjectivities are constructed and those constructions are disseminated by population programs and women's NGOs. That is to say, I cannot assess as to what extent these subjectivities actually have or have not been incorporated into, for instance, local women's NGO projects, national family planning consultancy, or public health services, or have become hegemonic on the local or at the level of the individuals as such. Such an assessment would require further research (see Pühl/Schultz 2001).

The Cairo Programme of Action established the concept of individual reproductive rights and reproductive health in population policies and placed the main focus on women's self-determination and empowerment (UN 1994). In so doing, it replaced the programmatic subjects of the pre-Cairo era, who had usually been seen as passive "acceptors" of family planning programs, with an active individual autonomously managing his or her "reproductive behavior" and "reproductive health." While in the post-Cairo era the demographic target of reducing global population growth has taken a back seat as far as the concrete level of actual programs is concerned, it has nevertheless remained the motivational and strategic centerpiece of the population policies regime. Thus, in global population policy, the difference between voluntariness and coercion, between body politics and popu-

---

7   Exceptions are Hartmann 1995; 2002; Rao 2004; Rao/Sexton 2010 and Silliman/Bhattarcharjee 2002.

lation politics, and between demographic planning and individual health management *is,* in fact, blurry. However, rather than neglecting the dimension of a demographic rationale altogether and opposing old and new biopolitics, in my view, we should scrutinize the specific articulations between state-based demographic rationalities and these new subjectivities.

In the following, I will document the continuities as well as the "postcatastrophic" transformations of the post-Cairo demographic strategies and add some theoretical remarks concerning demographic knowledge and the conceptualization of biopolitical statehood. Second, I will present a brief introduction to the changes on the micro-level, that is, the individualized and gendered subjectivities in the post-Cairo era. Third, I will demonstrate the analytical gain from analyzing the articulations of population policies and body policies. The discussion will focus particularly on the relevance of health rationales as the central link of this articulation. I will conclude with some theses regarding the debate on current biopolitics.

The project of international policies aimed at reducing global population growth can be traced back to the time period following World War II when private industrial foundations in the United States and representatives of eugenic and birth control movements that had formerly been confined to the national level started forming a network of think tanks, demographic research centers, lobby groups, and family planning organizations (Gordon 1977). Since the mid-1960s, these organizations have managed to establish their political project in US development policies and since the late 1960s in multilateral organizations, such as the United Nations Population Fund (UNFPA), in the population offices of the World Health Organization (WHO), and the World Bank (Donaldson 1990). Later, development ministries in European countries and Japan joined this project, too. In social science, "population establishment" has become an established concept denoting this continually expanding network of institutions (Hartmann 1995). At first in Asian and Latin American and later in African countries, the population establishment initiated national institution-building processes and accomplished a rise in the number of national governments pursuing anti-natalist programs–from 49 in 1976 to 76 in 1996 (UN 1998). These national settings developed in heterogeneous ways. They ranged from repressive population programs of state bureaucracies, with clear targets in regard to the number of sterilizations to be carried out or long-term contraceptives to be distributed, to family planning programs, kept in a more liberal tone, in cooperation with private organizations or within the framework of public health systems in countries where governments felt more reluctant to adopt the neo-Malthusian rationale (Hartmann 1995; WEDO 1999). Furthermore, international population policies started as isolated programs of "contraceptive inundation" in the 1950s and 1960s (Warwick 1982: 85) but developed into more integrated policies based on multifaceted sociotechnocratic approaches. Those policies, however, basically boiled down to implementing contraceptive technologies via systems of "incentives/ disincentives" (Mass 1976; Schultz 2006: 100f).

Despite the heterogeneity of constellations and actors, various analyses have shown that the population establishment developed as a quite stable "closed network" (McNicoll 1994: 657) for several reasons: it developed as a global experts pool with common codes and a revolving door system of employment in the various programs (Heim/Schaz 1996: 153), and was also tied together by joint funding sources. Most of all, the population establishment is a knowledge network that was kept together by the joint project of expounding the problems of population growth as a source of social crisis and proposing joint strategies of reducing it (Demeny 1988). The presupposition of population growth–always referring to poor populations in the South–as an a priori problematic development (Furedi 1997) essentially remained uncontested whereas the particular social crises that were attributed to it changed over time. In the early days of the population establishment's activities, population growth was said to cause "political instability" and excess consumption of resources in the (ex-)colonies; in the 1970s poverty and in the 1980s environmental destruction and migration were all considered consequences of too many people populating the globe.

Since the UN conference in Cairo, however, the population establishment has played down its population policy goals and pretends to have replaced them with goals of promoting individual reproductive rights and women's health. This conclusion, however, is misleading. It is at odds with the spirit of the Cairo Programme of Action itself, which declares demographic objectives a legitimate part of national planning and international development policies and dedicates whole chapters to constructing demographic problems (UN 1994). Also, the actual direction of the international population programs refutes the assertion that anti-natalist demographic objectives have been abandoned.

Population stabilization remained an explicit core goal of the family planning programs of USAID (United States Agency for International Development) after Cairo, the most potent international donor to population programs (USAID 2005). Likewise, the second most important donor, the World Bank, declared "population stabilization" a still "unfinished agenda" of its work in the health, nutrition, and population sector (World Bank 2005). Certainly since Cairo, many governments in the South (mainly in Asia) have abandoned the pursuit of so-called targets, that is, specific national objectives for the number of sterilizations to be carried out and long-term contraceptives to be distributed in a certain time period. Nevertheless, raising the "contraceptive prevalence rate" (the ratio of women either married or in stable relationships who or whose partners use some sort of "modern" contraceptive technology) and lowering the "total fertility rate" (the average number of children per woman) remained the criteria for success (ARROW 1999; Schultz 2006: 193f; WEDO 1999). Moreover, the distribution of contraceptives and sterilizations remained an important target of population policy funding although it has ceased to be the main focus of the population budgets because, since Cairo, HIV/AIDS and maternal health programs have been incorporated into the population budgets (see UNFPA 2009).

In addition, the large population agencies still put an emphasis on sterilizations and long-term contraceptives (WEDO 1999). For instance, in the post-Cairo period, the UNFPA distributed 100,000 units of the hormone implant Norplant in the country receiving the most international funding, Bangladesh, along with instructions for the providing NGOs to refrain from surgically removing the implants from women before five years had passed (interview Huq, women's rights organization Naripokkho Bangladesh, 2/7/ 1999; WEDO 1999). Promoting contraceptives that are controlled by the providers and have a long-term effect is common practice in international programs in order to minimize "discontinuation rates" and maximize "couple years of protection."

Last but not least, there have been cases of repressive practices in population programs, even in the post-Cairo period. To a significant extent, those cases include the countries that receive the most international funding. Thus, in several focus countries of Asian population policies (Bangladesh, India, Indonesia), extortion practices have persisted in form of making welfare benefits contingent on the participation in sterilization or contraceptives programs or by offering "compensation" payments for sterilization (WEDO 1999). Some Indian states have deprived parents with more than two children the right to be elected to local councils or have denied their children admission to federal schools (Mukherjee 2002; Rao 2010). Likewise, the case of Peru, the recipient of the most international funding among the Latin American countries in the second half of the 1990s, exemplifies the motives and dynamics of international population policies: the Peruvian Fujimori government implemented a national reproductive health program in 1996-98 leading to the sterilization of 300,000 persons and employed a host of measures of various sorts based on coercion, pressure, and extortion. Thus, the health system's employees were to report a certain number of sterilizations per month or else face dismissal; in the Andean highlands "tubal ligation festivals" took place where women were offered sterilization in exchange for a free hair-do or dental care; food aid and treatment in health centers were made contingent on the consent to sterilization, and there were even cases of women being locked up and coerced into surgery (Barthélemy 2004; CLADEM 1999; Schultz 2000; 2006).

Admittedly, this first glance at post-Cairo population policies is not to belie the changes brought about by the Cairo process. On the level of macro-demographic knowledge production, these changes can be summarized as the beginning of a post-catastrophic period (see Schultz 2006: 183-188). The apocalyptic propaganda of the 1980s and early 1990s, predicting a "population explosion" in the near future and stressing the failure of previous regulations, thus calling for increased investments in "saving the planet," made room for a more lenient vocabulary, avoiding concepts like "surplus population." After Cairo, the population establishment presented its own history as one shaped by success, claiming credit for the global decrease in birth rates in recent decades (Bongaarts/Sinding 2009). It developed more complex strategies of problematizing demographic development and adopted a more flexible intervention repertoire.

The emphasis was no longer on population growth as the single cause of manifold crisis phenomena but on the construction of a cybernetic problem according to which population growth is framed both as a condition for and a result of different social problems and crises and is also combined with other factors. Demographic analysis is now differentiated along different factors, target groups, and country settings. For instance, after Cairo, the population establishment has emphasized the "unwanted fertility" problem in some countries, for example in Latin America, resulting from the statistical difference between the reported number of desired children and the actual number of children. In others, above all in Sub-Saharan countries, the focus mostly remained on the supposedly too high "wanted fertility" or "desired family size" (without ever considering how this collides with the concept of freedom of choice). In countries with a strong decrease of birth rates in recent decades, the population establishment, in turn, prioritized the "population momentum" in anti-natalist policies (Bongaarts 1994; interview Merrick, World Bank, 9/15/1999; World Bank 2007a; 2007b). The term "population momentum" refers to the prognosis that today's numerous generations of adolescents, who were born in a time of high fertility, generate demographic growth effects even if they have only few children themselves. In some countries, delaying birth to a time later in life therefore became the slogan to attenuate this demographic effect (Speidel 2009; UNFPA 1999).

On the basis of this knowledge production, the World Bank developed concepts of demographic phases and country-specific measure mixes, thus continuing to place emphasis on a broad "contraceptive inundation" in some countries while developing strategies for specific, not yet sufficiently addressed target groups–such as rural populations, adolescents, and the unmarried–in other countries (interview Merrick, World Bank, 9/15/1999; World Bank, 2007a; 2007b).

The analysis and differentiation of national populations' age structures has become a special programmatic focus since the turn of the millennium. This focus shows that the population establishment has rehabilitated economic explanations. In the 1980s and 1990s, it had dissociated itself from the idea of a causal link between economic development and population growth due to a lack of evidence (see Cassen 1994)–and also because of the failure of catch-up development as the aim of development policies. However, after Cairo, the UNFPA again circulated calculations about a so-called "demographic bonus." In a phase of transition, the concept of a "demographic bonus" suggests that former high-fertility countries can achieve temporary economic gains when birth rates are decreasing while the effect of an "aging" population has not yet set in (UNFPA 2000; 2002).

DEMOGRAPHIC KNOWLEDGE AND NEO-MALTHUSIAN POLICY AS A STATE PROJECT

What do these post-Cairo developments indicate with regard to a biopolitical, state-led administration of populations? The thesis of the nation state being increasingly superseded and/or supplemented by global market-driven bioeconomic relations is misleading with regard to the story of population policies. As has been briefly outlined introduced above, international population policies have taken the opposite trajectory: from an international network of private actors towards a process of national institution-building. This transformation occurred through two often simultaneous but not identical processes: the adoption of anti-natalist policies by development bureaucracies in the donor countries and national institution-building in the area of population policies in the "subaltern" countries of the South. Thus, what we see is the concurrence of internationalization and nationalization in population policies rather than an increasing trend towards global networks and purely economic relationships. In order to account for the immense significance that private organizations and NGOs have had from the very beginning in the allocation of population policy funding, it seems appropriate to draw on neo-Marxist theories and Antonio Gramsci in speaking of an expanded and internationalized state (Borg 2001; Hirsch 2000). Referring to neo-Marxist theoretical perspectives, the project of global population policies can be conceptualized as inherently state-based not because of the complex network of actors or institutions involved but because they analyze the state as a form or as a condensation of power relations within society (Poulantzas 2004). Under this conceptual premise, the project of global population policies is per se a state project because the underlying demographic knowledge and the political project of neo-Malthusianism in themselves are bound to the state form: the project of population regulation establishes a specific social relationship within which social issues become translated into population issues and can thus be operationalized, which is not conceivable without the state form. Demography per se is a state science: fundamentally, it is based on statistical correlations between the population as an abstract quantity, as it is nationally measured by the state's statistics bureaus (and possibly aggregated to continental or global data sets afterwards), on the one hand, and on quantitative data about social living conditions, on the other (Heim/Schaz 1996; Hummel 2000).

These statistical correlations form the basis for the neo-Malthusianism idea that social crisis situations are caused by an imbalance between the population as "biomass," on the one hand, and limited resources, on the other. Within this paradigm, the population functions as a variable that has to be adjusted to the quantity of available resources whereas issues of redistribution and conditions of production are systematically excluded from this calculation.

From this point of view, every social problem can be formulated and operationalized as a population problem and dealt with in terms of socio-technocratic strategies. Thus, the neo-Malthusian project rests upon the utilitarian assumption that we can and should adjust a construct named "population surplus" to some quantity of available resources. Furthermore, neo-Malthusianism is essential to the project of global population control in that it gives the "surplus population"–the product of calculating average quantities–a concrete face through identifying the population group that would represent this excess quantity. The critical saying "fighting the poor instead of poverty" captures this mechanism quite well; the point of neo-Malthusianism is to declare exactly those people to be "superfluous" who already *are* excluded from access to social resources, work opportunities, or cultivable land. Bearing in mind the historical links to eugenics, the racism of the neo-Malthusian project in this respect is less in terms of a eugenic project of quality improvement than in denying the ecologically, economically, and/or socially excluded population the right to reproduce (and in that way questioning their very right to existence) for the sake of "life on the planet." The Foucauldian understanding of modern racism as an act of selection and a condition that makes it possible to justify acts of extermination in terms of optimizing life in general accurately captures the racist core of neo-Malthusianism. This analysis shows that modern biopolitics need not necessarily be about the superiority or inferiority of bodies or of "a people" but that racism can be anchored in demographic knowledge that ascribes social conditions of living to the people living under these conditions as permanent attributes or characteristics and in that sense to the bodies of the population groups concerned. Thus, the utilitarian and racist dimensions of today's expanded and internationalized biopolitical state principally remain in place even in post-Cairo, post-catastrophic population policies–albeit differentiated, fragmented, and multiplied through the complexity of demographic factors. This is a dimension of current biopolitics the analysis of which requires a radical deconstruction of demographic thinking and a more complex concept of the state.

The celebrated "paradigm shift" of Cairo did not affect the core motive of the population policy paradigm as outlined above. It is not class or race but gender relations that the post-Cairo population programs explicitly have addressed as the primary social category. However, while the concepts of individual reproductive rights, reproductive health, and empowerment have been moved to the fore, the old paradigm still lingers in the background. The new concepts have formed the framework for new individualized and gendered "programmatic subjectivities" in the post-Cairo era–be it the teen-ager who does not protect herself against pregnancy or sexually transmitted diseases, be it the victim of domestic violence who suffers a higher risk of maternal mortality, or be it the empowered woman who adequately "times" and "spaces" her pregnancies (Schultz 2006).

In order fully to understand the Cairo process, I have argued elsewhere that we have to consider the impact women's health movements had on this process (Schultz 2010). These movements built an international network in the mid-1980s to position the demand for self-determination and reproductive rights against the state-led regulation of populations, the "overpopulation myth," and human rights violations in the context of family planning programs. During the run-up to the Cairo UN conference in the early 1990s, however, "pragmatic" voices within women's NGOs' gained influence who were in favor of a strategy of dialogue with the population establishment in order to include gender and health issues in the framework of population policies. This strategy was successful in that the Cairo Programme of Action as result of the UN ICPD conference 1994 charters reproductive rights as "basic right(s) of all couples and individuals to decide freely and responsibly the number, spacing and timing of their children and to have the information and means to do so" (para. 7.3., UN 1994). Additionally, the document rebuffed the "incentives" and "targets" strategies, the basis of manifold human rights violations in the history of family planning programs, although it did so rather half-heartedly (para. 7.12., UN 1994).

The post-Cairo focus on a more complex understanding of gender also changed the way in which the population debate addressed social factors affecting individual "reproductive behavior." In the pre-Cairo era, the relation between macro-economic conditions and individual "behavior" used to be framed in terms of a simplistic model of women's social status. This model assumed that socioeconomic factors, such as women's education, income, and employment, conditioned women's decision to have more or fewer children. In the Cairo debate on gender, previously marginalized aspects came to the fore, like power relations in couple and family relationships, domestic violence, sexuality, and specific cultural beliefs about masculinity and femininity. Thus, an effort was made to establish a more comprehensive and complex understanding of reproduction that pays attention to cultural context and complex gender relations (Krause 2006). This new approach accounted for policy programs that addressed issues such as domestic violence and "male responsibility." Additionally, the question of sexual rights and health–strongly boosted by anti-HIV/AIDS policies–increasingly became the focal point of population policies' programmatic conceptions.

Empowerment, the central concept of the Cairo agenda, also points in the same direction: the Cairo Programme of Action calls for empowering women in terms of a broad range of social and cultural factors in order to improve their decision-making capacities about sexuality and reproduction, again under the premise that women's empowerment, although defined as an end in itself, also correlates with a decline in birth rates (UN 1994; see Hodgson/Watkins 1997).

Another concept that is also based on the demands of feminist movements and had a strong impact on the emergence of new individualized and activated programmatic subjectivities in population policies is the holistic "reproductive health" approach. In the Cairo Programme of Action, it is closely linked to the concept of reproductive rights, defined as "a state of complete physical, mental and social well-being" with regard to sexuality and reproduction (para. 7.2., UN 1994). The background to this concept was the women's health movements' critique that family planning programs often ignored the adverse health effects of modern contraceptives and sterilization methods for the sake of program effectiveness. First and foremost, however, the concept of reproductive health formed a response to the critique that population programs had separated the question of contraception from other women's health issues, thus effectively reducing women's health to contraception.

In their evaluation of the post-Cairo era, women's health NGOs have appraised the reproductive health concept as the most successful feminist concept within population policies (see for example WEDO 1999). It is true that in some places there was only a "semantic reform" and the previous population programs simply resurfaced in the guise of renamed reproductive health programs (DAWN 1999). In most cases, however, these reforms were indeed accompanied by increased funding to include other women's health services beyond family planning, albeit, as hinted above, as additional, secondary program elements. In this context, the production of epidemiological knowledge has expanded within the framework of post-Cairo discourse. Manifold reproductive and sexual risks have been identified and have formed the basis for identifying new target groups of population policies, differentiated especially along age groups, different sexual practices, and health status.

How can the complex micro-level scenario of the post-Cairo era, which we have covered briefly, be related to the demographic rationalities brought up before? Have concepts such as individual rights, empowerment, or reproductive health pushed these rationalities back or–as the pro-Cairo women NGO lobby has interpreted it–at least made them "immaterial," that is to say without noticeable effects in practice at the level of the concrete programs (Finkle/McIntosh 1994: 25)?

THE ARTICULATION OF DEMOGRAPHY, GENDER, AND HEALTH CONCEPTS

In my view, an analysis of articulation can explain why gender policy concepts could be established so successfully that some have described the Cairo Programme of Action as the "most feminist document" among all UN policies of the 1990s (Tinker 1999). I hold that these changes cannot simply be explained in terms of a changed balance of power between the population establishment and women's health movements, for in the mid-1990s the project of reducing population growth was not facing a crisis. On the contrary, it was very much on the rise; it had continually been expanding both institutionally and financially since the 1960s and had been established in "developing countries" by national institution-building, as demonstrated above. Moreover, thanks to the ecology movements and their construction of the global population as a strain on the planet's carrying capacity, global population programs had received additional legitimization. Steven Sinding, renowned expert of the population establishment, who is considered one of the architects of the Cairo process, once explained the successes of gender concepts this way (Sinding 2000): the "why" of global population growth control no longer was an issue of contention in the 1990s because the anti-natalist project for the most part had been established globally. Thus, during and after Cairo, debates about the "how" of population policies prevailed. The success of gender policy concepts has to be linked to this focus on the "how": body politics and the social conditions of individual reproductive behavior came to the fore, with gender relations providing an important context for understanding them, while macro-demographic criteria defining more or less desirable populations–basically linked to the categories class and race–took a back seat.

This takes us to the question whether and in what way the new concepts were actually functional in promoting demographic goals and how these goals were sustained and reformulated on the micro-political level. In order to answer these questions, I will analyze the gender policy concepts with regard to whether and to what degree they imply an "anti-natalist bias." This bias may comprise a focus on reducing pro-natalist social coercion of women rather than on the analysis and critique of anti-natalist combinations or on incentives for practicing individual birth control rather than on improving the living conditions of women with children. An anti-natalist bias may also consist in establishing certain norms about how pregnancies should be planned, "spaced," and "timed."

The concepts of reproductive rights and empowerment, both referring to women's individual autonomy with respect to sexuality and the decision of whether to have children or not, have been shaped in a specific way in the context of post-Cairo policies: reproductive rights had been the central point of reference of the international women's health movement that had emerged as a protest movement in the 1980s. In the context of this movement, and in opposition against global population policies, reproductive rights were framed in such a comprehensive way that they included the right to abortion and contraception as well as the "right to reproduce" (interview Nair, Women's Global Network for Reproductive Rights, 2/19/2001; Bradish/Feyerabend/Winkler 1989). They were largely constructed as defensive rights, directed against the population policy project, violent or oppressive forms of control over women's bodies, and threats against self-determination. Furthermore, the concept of reproductive rights, as promoted by the international women's health movement at that time, understood rights in terms of collective claims rather than universal norms or legislative standards. The movement thereby avoided establishing general criteria for an adequate reproductive "behavior" or for the proper use of reproductive rights on an individual level. Furthermore, the concept of reproductive rights was articulated to broader debates over the gender-based division of labor, social organization of child care, and sexual politics, thus addressing reproduction and its social context as a broader political issue that cannot be reduced to individual reproductive decision-making (Schultz 2006: 120-126).

In post-Cairo policies, however, reproductive rights have turned into something different. An increasingly institution- and state-oriented community of professionalized women's NGOs sees them as a universal, legal canon of more or less binding documents of international law and national legal projects (CRLP 2000). In exceptional cases of extreme human rights violations, NGOs specialized in law, actually have used this canon to combat repressive practices in population programs (CLADEM 1999). However, the classic notion of reproductive rights as defensive rights has become rather marginal in post-Cairo policies, both with regard to the population establishment and the large pro-Cairo women's NGOs. The main focus has become the interpretation of reproductive rights as rights that grant access to certain health services, particularly the supply of contraceptives. In the formulation of the Cairo Programme of Action, individuals are supposed to decide "freely and responsibly the number, spacing and timing of their children" (para. 7.3, UN 1994). In the population programs, self-determined and responsible behavior generally is interpreted as using modern contraceptives, planning children, not having children before the age of 18 and after the age of 35, keeping an appropriate distance between births ("birth spacing"), and avoiding "reproductive risks." Thus, this conceptualization of reproductive rights as rights of access implies a model of self-responsibility and self-determination that is normatively charged and establishes an anti-natalist bias with respect to the proper form of decision-making.

Likewise, the individualizing perspective on reproductive rights of the post-Cairo period implies that the political critique of technology voiced by feminist movements before Cairo has largely lost ground. The paradigms of informed consent and freedom of choice concerning contraceptive methods (also referred to as "cafeteria approach") are certainly useful in criticizing repressive measures. However, these approaches fail to grasp the more general questions raised by the critique of technology, such as why certain methods are invented and distributed or why certain contraceptives or sterilization techniques are preferred with respect to specific populations. These questions have become largely marginalized in the post-Cairo era.

While the concept of reproductive rights nevertheless has remained politically ambivalent–since it is still applied in non-repressive ways from time to time–the empowerment concept probably has formed the decisive link between the micro-political level of individual bodies and behavior with a demographic rationale directed at the population (Könninger 2001). The basic assumption of the Cairo consensus that individual empowerment of women in the South would by default lead to a decrease of birth rates implied a culturalizing perspective on gender hierarchies (Krause 2006). By this I mean that the "Third World woman" is perceived as being restricted by "traditional," "patriarchal," or "fundamentalist" structures, particularly regarding her position within the family or a relationship, and having children is considered a particularly aggravating factor in this respect. Thus, pro-natalist policies or social conditions that foster large families are viewed as "disabling conditions" whereas anti-natalist pressures of different sorts, if considered at all, have been conceived as working in the right direction. The shift from an emphasis on socio-economic context to culturalizing approaches to individual reproductive behavior was in line with a general paradigm shift in developmental theory in the past decades from a focus on socio-economic macro-conditions to micro-sociological reflections about cultural habits and institutions (see Escobar 1995).

Furthermore, the post-Cairo empowerment concept has indicated that self-determination, understood as the ability to control one's reproductive behavior according to one's own interests, no longer serves as the starting point of policies but, conversely, appears as the result of biopolitical intervention. In this sense, the empowerment concept has produced an abundance of ascriptions attributed to the supposedly disempowered subjects as well as manifold political strategies enabling them to enhance their decision-making capacities in a certain direction (see Cruikshank 1999). This reverse effect of the empowerment concept was exemplified quite clearly by how the UNFPA measured self-determination in its world population report published in the year of the Cairo conference: the report presented statistics on women's average age at marriage and at giving birth for the first time for three countries, commenting that from this data one could read the status of women's freedom of choice in the respective country (UNFPA 1994: 13). In this sense, empowerment seemed to be predestined for reformulating and reinstating demographic objectives at the level of individual norms of behavior.

So far, I have argued that the concepts of reproductive rights and empowerment in post-Cairo discourse offered a general frame for articulating feminist concepts with anti-natalist norms of reproductive behavior. However, these concepts did not provide detailed quantitative criteria for establishing by what standard and at what time which category of women should not have (additional) children. The field of epidemiological knowledge has offered a variety of starting points for such fine-tuning (Schultz 2003). I hold that these opportunities of epidemiological knowledge production explain why and how women's health issues were able to evolve into a central field of knowledge production and a key area for the self-presentation of the post-Cairo population establishment such that a specific epidemiological medicalization of international population policies could take place (Qadeer 1998).

Reproductive risk prevention policies are very suitable tools for anti-natalist strategies in that, from an epidemiological standpoint, it appears clear that it is more beneficial and less risky to a woman's health *not* to become pregnant than to become pregnant. After all, a woman who avoids pregnancy is not confronted with "reproductive risks," let alone with the possibility of dying due to its consequences. Hence, maternal mortality has formed the main focal point of the expanding epidemiological knowledge of the post-Cairo era. For example, the German state's development agency Society for Technical Cooperation (GTZ) celebrated the tenth anniversary of the Cairo conference in 2004 together with the openly neo-Malthusian NGO German World Population Foundation (DSW) by launching a campaign for "Safe Motherhood." This and other campaigns against maternal mortality refer to the fact that every year 500,000 women, 99 percent of whom live in the "developing countries," die in the course of a pregnancy, particularly during birth but also in the aftermath of abortion complications (World Bank 1999b: 5). The Safe Motherhood Initiative, which was started in 1987 by the large agencies of the population establishment, at first focused on broad social, political, and preventive strategies (for example, risk screening in antenatal programs) of fighting maternal mortality (Starrs

1987). At the end of the 1990s, however, the population establishment admitted the failure of this strategy. The agencies declared that the lack of healthcare infrastructure was a significant cause of maternal mortality and that a well-developed, area-wide emergency obstetric care system together with safe abortion facilities were more appropriate means of helping women "once pregnant" (Starrs 1997). After all, most complications during birth cannot be predicted or prevented on an individual level but can easily be treated (see Maine 2000). Despite this concession, which principally questions preventive strategies as an appropriate approach to fight maternal mortality, the population establishment continued to direct its attention (and most of its members' investments) to policies targeting maternal mortality on a level of prevention. The prevention of (risk) pregnancies became the main focus of attention.

Prevention of "reproductive risks" is a paradigm on the basis of which the population establishment has identified a variety of risk regions, risk groups, and risk factors in order to determine which women at what age in which situations face an increased risk of maternal mortality. Drawing on that data, the population agencies launched specific family planning programs for these groups. Since the beginning of the new millennium, the pregnant adolescent has become the shooting star among the new subjects at risk. Yet, the fact is that the difference between adolescent and adult women's maternal mortality risk due to abortion or birth complications is many times lower than the difference of such risk between women in richer and poorer countries.[8] Nevertheless, programs for preventing teenage pregnancies form a link between demographic strategies and epidemiological parameters. In this context, demographic rationales are decisive as to when and where the focus is directed at "adolescents' reproductive health." UNFPA, USAID, and the World Bank all state that the prevention of teenage pregnancies is particularly pressing in those countries where the demographic effect of population momentum could be counteracted by delaying

---

8   In 2004, a UNFPA report explained that in West Africa the risk of a woman to die from the consequences of pregnancy or birth is 1 in 12 while in more developed regions of the world it is 1 in 4000 (UNFPA 2004b: 67). The Safe Motherhood Initiative agencies calculated the difference between the maternal mortality risk of an adolescent between age 15 and 19 as twice that of a woman between 20 and 29 (Starrs 1997: 20).

birth within those age groups who were born during periods of higher fertility and who are now "entering reproductive age" in large numbers.

The World Bank, for instance, in its post-Cairo programs, has considered the focus on adolescents particularly important in countries with a considerable decrease in birth rates in recent decades, for example India and Bangladesh. Contrary to this, the "country method mix" in several Sub-Saharan countries continued to focus on the distribution of family planning methods to adults (World Bank 1999a). Thus, we can conclude that the new micro-demographic programmatic subjectivities of the post-Cairo population policies have been activated particularly at times when and in regions where they were matching corresponding macro-demographic strategies. Although the primary motive for placing adolescents at the center of population policies was a demographic one in post-Cairo programs, the various instruments to prevent teenage pregnancies can be described as differentiated security technologies. That means that the population establishment has combined emancipatory projects that focus on sexual education and the adolescents' right of individual access to contraceptives–supported by feminist NGOs–with strategies of sexual abstinence informed by traditional conservative values and with legal strategies of raising the age of consent to marriage, depending on which sexual practices have been found to be prevalent among adolescents in certain regions or settings (see Starrs 1997: 21; UNFPA 2004a: 92). Thus, it were not universal human rights for adolescents or general sexual moral standards that have been at the heart of concern of these post-Cairo population policy schemes but the question as to which strategies were most promising in order to achieve anti-natalist objectives in specific situations.

CONCLUSIONS

What does the articulation between demographic objectives and gender policies reveal about a supposedly new regime of global biopolitics? I have shown that the new "programmatic subjectivities" of population policies after Cairo have indeed placed an individual who is responsible for his or her own health at the center of attention, and that this shift was reflected in the paradigms of self-determination and empowerment. However, the dynamics, the success, and the specific shape of these subjectivities cannot be fully understood without considering their articulation with demographic goals still prevalent in international health and development policies after Cairo. The account presented here differs in two respects from the analysis of a new biopolitics found in governmentality studies.

Firstly, I have argued that the international demographic project cannot be comprehended without analyzing the expanded and internationalized biopolitical state, which has remained focused on the management of neatly circumscribed populations on the basis of neo-Malthusian crisis interpretations, albeit the underlying notion of a population has increasingly been differentiated along several demographic factors after Cairo. The primary functional principle of the international demographic project is still to define certain population groups as economically or ecologically superfluous. Thus, we can still speak of a management of concrete populations by the state(s); a management that cannot be reduced to the production of diffuse "dividuals" on the basis of epidemiological risk technologies (see Lemke 2000). Nevertheless, epidemiological risks provide an important vehicle for reformulating demographic objectives indirectly on the basis of health rationales. In order to reveal the still prevalent neo-Malthusian motives of current development policies, we need to develop a critique of demography. This critique has to address not only policies directed at curbing global population growth but also the rehabilitation of demographic knowledge in the "advanced liberal societies of the West," where knowledge these days is being mobilized for pro-natalist purposes, for legitimizing the cutback of welfare systems, or for the objectives of migration control and regulation (Baureithel 2007).

Secondly, as opposed to Rose, I emphasize that the population policies' new "programmatic subjectivities" cannot be understood with regard to their liberal, activating, and scope-expanding nature only. Especially considering postcolonial perspectives and the conservative essence of the neo-Malthusian rationale in wanting to adapt the population as a variable to the societal status quo, the problematic structure of the empowerment discourse needs to be highlighted. This structure is rooted in the wish to control "other" women and their "reproductive behavior," constructing them as disempowered and thus employing the concept of self-determination for normative biopolitical interventions. Ulrich Bröckling once spoke of the "appealing if not prescriptive" nature of the neoliberal interpellation of the self-responsible individual (Bröckling 2001: 5). My suggestion is to consider "appealing" and "prescriptive" not as gradual differences on the same scale but as a constitutive difference based on social hierarchies. While some people are considered as endowed with a potential for self-determination that simply needs to be invoked, others are constructed as incapable of self-determination, thus needing to be educated, pressed, or, paradoxically, even coerced into self-determination. The Peruvian sterilization program is testimony to the fact that the call for women to "take matters into their own hands," as was proclaimed by the Peruvian president Fujimori at the launch of his reproductive health program, can easily go along with repressive measures. In order to understand the hierarchy between appealing and prescriptive interpellations inscribed into the new subjectivities, I refer to the concept of intersectionality,[9] denoting the intertwinement of different lines of social hierarchization, such as gender, race, and class. This aspect, in my view, is rather neglected in governmentality studies, which leads to the supposedly unintended but somewhat inevitable effect of reifying, albeit critically, the idea of a neutral autonomous liberal individual.

Looking at the intertwined inscription of race, gender, and class into new subjectivities is also instructive if we want to comprehend mechanisms of depoliticization. The predominance of individualized gender concepts in post-Cairo policies supports the prevalence of micro-political "how" questions concerning reproduction policies in that micro-demographic knowledge focuses on the question of how gender influences individual reproductive decision-making. Thus, the focus on gender as an isolated category in the post-Cairo era glosses over the utilitarian premises and the lines of hierarchy along race and class that are still operative with regard to the "why" of population regulations on the macro-level.

Finally, as regards the concept of biopolitics, these two arguments lead me to the following conclusion: in order not to reify the post-Cairo population agenda, which obscures, detaches, and depoliticizes the macro-level of population management, we should keep in mind the selective dimension of biopolitics pointed out by Foucault. I think it is important to remember that Foucault understood biopolitics in the context of the liberal, individualizing management of the population in the sense of governmentality. In my view,

---

9 In the Anglo-American debate, intersectionality has evolved as the main concept for analyzing the interdependency of different social patterns of hierarchization, often conceived as the triad of "race, class, and gender" (see Knapp 2005).

looking at the tension between self-technologies, individualization, and the production of subjectivities, on the one hand, and macro-political management, standardization, and racism, on the other, remains a useful conceptual foundation for the analysis of contemporary population and biopolitics, which we should not discard by historizing biopolitics.

REFERENCES

ARROW (Asian-Pacific Resource & Research Centre for Women) (1999): Changes in population policies and programmes post-ICPD Cairo: a regional research project. Overview of main findings, Kuala Lumpur.

Barthélémy, Francoise (2004): "Zwangssterilisation in Peru: Gut verkauft, schlecht gemeint," in: Le Monde Diplomatique, May 2004, pp. 18-19.

Baureithel, Ulrike (2007): "Baby-Bataillone. Demografisches Aufmarschgebiet: Von Müttern, Kinderlosen und der 'Schuld' der Emanzipation", in: Prokla, 146, pp. 25-37.

Bongaarts, John W. (1994): "Population policy options in the developing world," in: Science, 263, 2/11/1994, pp. 771-776.

Bongaarts, John W./Sinding, Steven (2009): "A response to critics of family planning programs," in: International Perspectives on Sexual and Reproductive Health, 35(1), pp. 39-44.

Borg, Erik (2001): Projekt Globalisierung. Soziale Konflikte im Konflikt um Hegemonie, Hanover: Offizin.

Bradish, Paula/Feyerabend, Erika/Winkler, Ute (eds) (1989): Frauen gegen Gen- und Reproduktionstechnologien. Beiträge zum 2. bundesweiten Kongreß in Frankfurt, 28-30 Oct 1988, Munich: Frauenoffensive.

Bröckling, Ulrich (2001): "Das unternehmerische Selbst und seine Geschlechter," paper presented at the symposium: Welcome to the Revolution 9-11 Nov 2001, Hochschule für Gestaltung und Kunst, Zurich.

Bröckling, Ulrich/Krasmann, Susanne/Lemke, Thomas (eds) (2000): Gouvernementalität der Gegenwart. Studien zur Ökonomisierung des Sozialen, Frankfurt a.M.: Suhrkamp.

Burchell, Graham (1993): "Liberal government and the techniques of the self," in: Economy and Society, 22(3): pp. 267-282.

Burchell, Graham/Gordon, Colin/Miller, Peter (1993): The Foucault effect. Studies in governmentality, Hemel Hempstead: Harvester Wheatsheaf.

Cassen, Robert (ed) (1994): Population and development: old debates, new conclusions, New Brunswick: Transaction Publishers.

CLADEM (Comité de America Latina y el Caribe para la Defensa de los Derechos de la Mujer) (1999): Nada personal. reporte de derechos humanos sobre la aplicación de la anticoncepción quirúrgica en el Perú, Lima: CLADEM.

CRLP (Center for Reproductive Law and Policy) (2000): Reproductive rights 2000. Moving forward, New York: CRLP.

Cruikshank, Barbara (1999): The will to empower. Democratic citizens and other subjects, Ithaca, London: Cornell University Press.

DAWN (Development Alternatives with Women for a New Era) (1999): Implementing ICPD: moving forward in the eye of the storm, DAWNs Platform for Cairo+5, January 1999, Suva: DAWN.

Demeny, Paul (1988): "Social science and population policy," in: Population and Development Review, 14 (3): pp. 451-479.

Donaldson, Peter J. (1990): Nature against us: The United States and the world population crisis 1965-1980, Chapel Hill/North Carolina/London: University of North Carolina Press.

Escobar, Arturo (1995): Encountering development. The making and unmaking of the Third World, Princeton: Princeton University Press.

Finkle, Jason/McIntosh, Alison (1994): "The new politics of population," in: Jason Finkle/Alison McIntosh (eds), The new politics of population. Conflict and consensus in family planning, New York: Population Council, pp. 3-34.

Foucault, Michel (1983): Der Wille zum Wissen. Sexualität und Wahrheit 1, Frankfurt a.M.: Suhrkamp.

— (2001): "Vorlesung 17. März 1976," in: Michel Foucault, In Verteidigung der Gesellschaft, Frankfurt a.M.: Suhrkamp, pp. 282-311.

— (2003): "Die Geburt der Biopolitik," in: Michel Foucault, Dits et Ecrits. Schriften. Dritter Band, Frankfurt a.M.: Suhrkamp, pp. 1020-1028.

— (2004): Geschichte der Gouvernementalität, Frankfurt a.M.: Suhrkamp.

Furedi, Frank (1997): Population and development, New York: St. Martins Press.

Gordon, Linda (1977): Women's body, women's right. A social history of birth control in America, New York: Viking.

Gutiérrez Rodríguez, Encarnación (2003): "Gouvernementalität und die Ethnisierung des Sozialen. Migration, Arbeit und Biopolitik," in: Marianne Pieper/Encarnación Gutiérrez Rodríguez (eds), Gouvernementalität. Ein sozialwissenschaftliches Konzept in Anschluss an Foucault, Frankfurt a.M./New York: Campus, pp. 161-178

Hartmann, Betsy (1995): Reproductive rights and wrongs. The global politics of population control, Boston: South End Press.

— (2002): "The changing faces of population control," in: Silliman/Bhattacharjee, Policing the national body. Race, gender, and criminalization, pp. 259-289.

Heath, Deborah/Rapp, Rayna/Taussig, Karen-Sue (2004): "Genetic citizenship," in: David Nugent/Joan Vincent (eds), A companion to the anthropology of politics, Malden/Oxford/Victoria: Blackwell Publishing, pp. 152-166.

Heim, Susanne/Schaz, Ulrike (1996): Berechnung und Beschwörung. Überbevölkerung–Kritik einer Debatte, Berlin: Schwarze Risse/Rote Straße.

Hirsch, Joachim (2000): "Die Internationalisierung des Staates", in: Das Argument, 236: pp. 325-340.

Hodgson, Dennis/Watkins, Susan Cotts (1997): "Feminists and neo-Malthusians past and present alliances," in: Population and Development Review, 23(3), pp. 469-523.

Hummel, Diana (2000): Der Bevölkerungsdiskurs. Demographisches Wissen und politische Macht, Opladen: Leske & Budrich.

Jahn, Thomas/Wehling, Peter (1998): "Gesellschaftliche Naturverhältnisse. Konturen eines theoretischen Konzepts," in: Karl-Werner Brand (ed), Soziologie und Natur. Theoretische Perspektiven, Opladen: Leske & Budrich, pp. 75-96.

Jessop, Bob (1990): State theory. Putting the capitalist state in its place, Cambridge: Polity Press.

Knapp, Gudrun-Axeli (2005): "Traveling Theories: Anmerkungen zur neueren Diskussion über 'Race, Class, and Gender'", in: Österreichische Zeitschrift für Geschichtswissenschaften, 16(1): pp. 88-110.

Könninger, Sabine (2001): Das Konzept des Women's Empowerment in der internationalen bevölkerungspolitischen Debatte, unpublished thesis, University of Hanover, Hanover.

Krause, Martina (2006): "Zwischen Vorurteilen und neuer Lebensphilosophie. Programme zur reproduktiven Gesundheit in Mexiko," in: Peripherie. Zeitschrift für Ökonomie und Politik in der Dritten Welt, 26, (101/102), pp. 166-190.

Laclau, Ernesto/Mouffe Chantal (1985): Hegemony and socialist strategy. Towards a radical democratic politics, London/New York: Verso.
Lemke, Thomas (2000): "Die Regierung der Risiken. Von der Eugenik zur genetischen Gouvernementalität," in: Ulrich Bröckling/Susanne Krasmann/Thomas Lemke (eds), Gouvernementalität der Gegenwart. Studien zur Ökonomisierung des Sozialen, Frankfurt a.M.: Suhrkamp.
— (2004): Veranlagung und Verantwortung. Genetische Diagnostik zwischen Selbstbestimmung und Schicksal, Bielefeld: transcript.
Maine, Deborah (2000): "What is so special about maternal mortality?", in: Marge Berer/T. K. Sundari Ravindran (eds), Safe motherhood initiatives: critical issues, special issue of Reproductive Health Matters, London: Blackwell Science, pp. 175-181.
Mass, Bonnie (1976): Population target. The political economy of population control in Latin America, Toronto: Latin American Working Group.
McNicoll, Geoffrey (1994): "Laurie Ann Mazur. Beyond the numbers. Book review," in: Population and Development Review, 20 (2): pp. 656-660.
Mukherjee, Vanita Nayak (2002): "Gender matters," paper presented at the Symposium on Population Planning and Advocacy, Delhi, July 2002, available at http://www.india-seminar.com/2002/511.htm (last accessed 2/7/2005).
O'Malley, Pat/Weir, Lorna/Shearing, Cllifford (1997): "Governmentality, criticism, politics," in: Economy and Society, 26(4): pp- 501-517.
OECD (2010): "Recent trends in official development assistance to health, update," available at: http://www.oecd.org/dataoecd/1/11/37461859.pdf (last accessed 11/30/2010).
Petchesky, Rosalind/Judd, Karen (1998): Negotiating reproductive rights. Women's perspectives across countries and cultures, London/New York: IRRRAG.
Poulantzas, Nicos (2004): Staatstheorie. Politischer Überbau, Ideologie, Hamburg: VSA.
Pühl, Katharina/Schultz, Susanne (2001): "Gouvernementalität und Geschlecht. Über das Paradox der Festschreibung und Flexibilisierung der Geschlechterverhältnisse," in: Sabine Hess/Ramona Lenz (eds), Geschlecht und Globalisierung, Königstein Taunus: Ulrike Helmer, pp. 102-127.

Qadeer, Imrana. (1998): "Reproductive health and rights. A public health perspective," in: Centre of Social Medicine and Community Health (ed), Reproductive health in India's primary health care, New Delhi: Jawaharlal Nehru University, 1-26.
Rabinow, Paul/Rose, Nikolas (2003): "Thoughts on the concept of biopower today," available at http://www.lse.ac.uk/collections/sociology/pdf/RabinowandRose-BiopowerToday03.pdf (last accessed 8/7/2005).
Rao, Mohan (2004): From population control to reproductive health. Malthusian arithmetic, New Delhi: Sage.
— (2010): "An entangled skein: neo-Malthusianisms in neo-liberal times," in: Rao/Sexton, Markets and Malthus. Population, gender, and health in neo-liberal times, pp. 103-126.
Rao, Mohan/Sexton, Sarah (eds) (2010): Markets and Malthus. Population, gender, and health in neo-liberal times, Delhi: Sage.
Rose, Nikolas (2001): "The politics of life itself," in: Theory, Culture and Society, 18 (66): pp. 1-30.
Rose, Nikolas/Novas, Carlos (2002): "Biological citizenship," available at: http://www2.lse.ac.uk/sociology/pdf/RoseandNovasBiologicalCitizenship2002.pdf (last accessed 1/12/2010).
Schultz, Susanne (2000): "Leise Diplomatie. Die Politik feministischer Nicht-Regierungsorganisationen zur Sterilisationskampagne in Peru," in: Karin Gabbert et al (eds), Geschlecht und Macht. Lateinamerika Jahrbuch 24, Analysen und Berichte, Münster: Westfälisches Dampfboot, pp. 55-65.
— (2003): "Von der Regierung reproduktiver Risiken. Gender und die Medikalisierung internationaler Bevölkerungspolitik," in: Marianne Pieper/Encarnacion Gutiérrez Rodríguez (eds), Gouvernementalität. Ein sozialwissenschaftliches Konzept in Anschluss an Foucault, Frankfurt a.M./New York: Campus, pp. 68-89.
— (2006): Hegemonie, Gouvernementalität, Biomacht. Reproduktive Risiken und die Transformation internationaler Bevölkerungspolitik, Münster: Westfälisches Dampfboot.
— (2010): "Redefining and medicalizing population policies: NGOs and their innovative contributions to the Post Cairo agenda," in: Rao/Sexton, Markets and Malthus, pp. 173-214.
Silliman, Jael/Bhattacharjee Annanya (eds) (2002): Policing the national body. Race, gender, and criminalization, Cambridge: South End Press.

Sinding, Steven (2000): "The great population debates. How relevant are they for the 21st century?" in: American Journal of Public Health, 90(12), pp. 1841-1845.

Speidel, Joseph et al (2009): "Population policies, programmes and the environment," in: Philosophical Transactions of the Royal Society, 364, pp. 3049-3065.

Starrs, Ann 1987: Preventing the tragedy of maternal deaths. A report on the International Safe Motherhood Conference in Nairobi/Kenia, Washington: World Bank.

— (1997): The safe motherhood action agenda. Priorities for the next decade, report on the Safe Motherhood Technical Consultation, 18-23 October 1997, Sri Lanka, New York: Inter-Agency Group for Safe Motherhood.

Tinker, Irene (1999): "Nongovernmental organizations. An alternative power base for women," in: Mary K. Meyer/Elisabeth Prügl (eds), Gender politics in global governance, Lanham/Boulder: Rowman & Littlefield Publishers, pp. 88-106.

UN (1994): Programme of Action of the International Conference on Population and Development. Report of the International Conference on Population and Development, 5-13 September 1994 in Cairo, New York, available at: http://www.unfpa.org/icpd/icpd_poa.htm (last accessed 5/9/2005).

— (1998): National population policies, New York: Department of Economic and Social Affairs Population Division/United Nations.

UNFPA (1994): Entscheidungsfreiheit und Verantwortung. Weltbevölkerungsbericht 1994, Bonn: Deutsche Gesellschaft für die Vereinten Nationen.

— (1999): A time between. Health, sexuality, and reproductive rights of young people, New York: UNFPA.

— (2000): Frauen und Männer–getrennte Welten? Weltbevölkerungsbericht 2000, Deutsche Stiftung Weltbevölkerung (ed), Stuttgart: Balance.

— (2002): Macroeconomics, poverty, population and development. The state of world population 2002, New York: UNFPA.

— (2004): Weltbevölkerungsbericht 2004, Deutsche Stiftung Weltbevölkerung (ed), Stuttgart: Balance.

— (2004b): Achieving the Cairo, Cairo+5 and Millennium Development Goals, New York: UNFPA.

— (2009): Financial resource flows for population activities 2007, New York: UNFPA.
USAID (2005): Family planning, available at: http://www.usaid.gov/our_work/global_health/pop/index.html (last accessed 7/13/2005).
Waldby, Catherine (2000): The visible human project, London: Routledge.
Warwick, Donald P. (1982): Bitter pills. Population policies and their implementation in eight developing countries, Cambridge/London/New York: Cambridge University Press.
WEDO (Women, Environment, and Development Organization) (1999): Risks, rights and reforms. A 50-country survey assessing government action five years after the International Conference on Population and Development, New York: WEDO.
World Bank (1999a): Population and the World Bank. Adapting to change, Human Development Network, Health, Nutrition, and Population Series. Washington D.C.: World Bank.
— (1999b): Safe motherhood and the World Bank, Human Development Network, Washington D.C.: World Bank.
— (2005): Population and reproductive health, available at: http://web.worldbank.org/ (last accessed 5/18/2005).
— (2007a): Healthy development. The World Bank strategy for HNP Results, April 2007, Washington D.C.: World Bank.
— (2007b): Population issues in the 21st century. The role of the World Bank, April 2007, Washington D.C.: World Bank.

List of Contributors

William Ray Arney has written on medicine, education and expertise. He is on the faculty of The Evergreen State College in Olympia, Washington USA.

Kathrin Braun is apl professor in Political Science at Leibniz University Hanover, Germany. Her research focuses on the emergence, transformation, and problematization of biopolitical modernist rationality in the politics of biomedicine, the politics of historic (in)justice, and political thought.

Svea L. Herrmann, Dr. phil., is postdoc researcher at Leibniz University Hanover, Germany. Her research interests refer to problematization processes in public policy debates and biopolitics and reparations politics. She is author of *Policy Debates on Reprogenetics. Problematisation of New Research in Great Britain and Germany* (Campus 2009). Her current research focuses on the politics of reparations for involuntary sterilisations.

Isabella Jordan, received her Dr. phil. in Political Science at Leibniz University Hanover, Germany (*Die Hospizbewegung in Deutschland und den Niederlanden. Palliativversorgung und Selbstbestimmung am Lebensende*, Campus 2007). She is postdoc researcher at the Department for Medical Ethics and History of Medicine, Göttingen. Her research focuses on hospice movements and palliative care, mercy killing debates, and eugenics.

Sabine Könninger studied Political Sciences and French. She is research assistant at the Institute of Economic Policy Research (Department of Economic Policy) at Karlsruhe Institute of Technology and doctoral student at

Leibniz University Hanover. Her current study is on the development, institutionalization and framing of bio- and nanoethicpolitics in France.

Helen Kohlen is junior professor of care policy and ethics at the Theological–Philosophical University of Vallendar in Germany and teaches at the faculty of nursing. In her current research she focuses on the transformations of care in psychiatry. She received her Dr. phil. in Political Science from Hanover University in 2008. Her work *Conflicts of Care* (Campus 2009) was awarded by the IMEW (*Institut Mensch Ethik Wissenschaft*).

Silja Samerski, Dr. phil., is assistant professor in the Department of Sociology at Leibniz University Hanover. She has a background in biology, philosophy, and social sciences. Her recent book is *Die Entscheidungsfalle. Wie genetische Aufklärung die Gesellschaft entmündigt* (Wissenschaftliche Buchgesellschaft 2010). Her current research focuses on the history and social function of professional counseling in managerial decision-making.

Marion Schumann received her Dr. phil. in Sociology from Leibniz University Hanover. Her doctoral thesis examines the history of midwifery in the Federal Republic of Germany (*Vom Dienst an Mutter und Kind zum Dienst nach Plan. Hebammen in der Bundesrepublik 1950-1975*, V&R unipress 2009). She works in the area of health promotion and self-help at the *Paritätischer Wohlfahrtsverband*, Hannover.

Susanne Schultz, Dr. phil., is a political scientist and postdoc researcher at Leibniz Universität Hanover and also editor for the Berlin based NGO *Gen-ethisches Netzwerk*. Her thesis focused on international population policies, state theory and the NGOization of women's health movements (*Hegemonie, Gouvernementalität, Biomacht. Reproduktive Risiken und die Transformation internationaler Bevölkerungspolitik*, Westfälisches Dampfboot 2006).